Behind the mirror

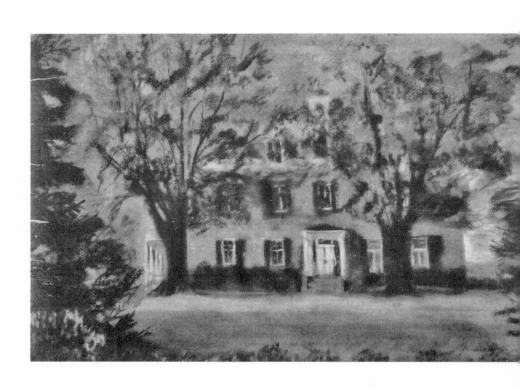

Behind the mirror

The story of a pioneer in autism treatment
and her work with children on the spectrum

Jeanne Simons

As told to and
with commentary by
Sabine Oishi, PhD

Foreword and Afterword by
James C. Harris, MD

Johns Hopkins University Press
Baltimore

Johns Hopkins University Press
2715 North Charles Street
Baltimore, Maryland 21218-4363
www.press.jhu.edu

Library of Congress Cataloging-in-Publication Data

Names: Simons, Jeanne, 1910–2005 author | Oishi, Sabine, 1934– author. |
    Harris, James C., author.
Title: Behind the mirror : The story of a pioneer in autism treatment
    and her work with children on the spectrum / Simons, Jeanne ;
    as told to and with commentary by Sabine Oishi, PhD ; foreword
    and afterword by James C. Harris, MD.
Description: Baltimore : Johns Hopkins University Press, 2021. | Includes
    bibliographical references.
Identifiers: LCCN 2020028520 | ISBN 9781421440767 (paperback) |
    ISBN 9781421440774 (ebook)
Subjects: LCSH: Simons, Jeanne—Health. | Autistic people—Biography. |
    Autism spectrum disorders—Patients—Rehabilitation. | Linwood
    Children's Center.
Classification: LCC RC553.A88 O46 2021 | DDC 616.85/882—dc23
LC record available at https://lccn.loc.gov/2020028520

A catalog record for this book is available from the British Library.

Frontispiece: Painting of the Linwood School by Jeanne Simons. Painting
was important to Jeanne throughout her life. Courtesy of the Linwood Center.

*Special discounts are available for bulk purchases of this book. For more information,
please contact Special Sales at specialsales@jh.edu.*

Johns Hopkins University Press uses environmentally friendly book materials,
including recycled text paper that is composed of at least 30 percent post-consumer
waste, whenever possible.

Jeanne Simons asked that this book be dedicated,

as was *The Hidden Child*, to the staff of the Linwood Center.

I would like to extend this dedication to everyone who,

like Jeanne, labors to help those most in need move toward

their utmost potential.

I had to defend against relationships at an early age to protect myself against the emotions of those around me. I had gone into hiding, both literally, under a table, and metaphorically, by disappearing behind a sort of one-way mirror inside my head that shielded my own thoughts from the intrusion of others but allowed me to observe them from a safe distance.

—Jeanne Simons

Contents

Illustrations appear following page 88

Foreword

Sabine Oishi's presentation of Jeanne Simons' life story is a revelation. Dr. Oishi, a developmental psychologist who studied with the renowned psychologist Jean Piaget, worked closely with Jeanne Simons for many years, coauthoring with her *The Hidden Child: The Linwood Method for Reaching the Autistic Child* (1). Jeanne entrusted Sabine with her life story, hoping it would be published. That hope has now come to fruition.

Jeanne Simons played an important role in the history of autism. It was Jeanne who convinced a skeptical Leo Kanner, the Johns Hopkins University child psychiatrist who first described early infantile autism in 1943, that these children—if sensitively engaged—could be treated. While Jeanne was working at Children's House in Washington, DC, as a child therapist in 1950, an eleven-year-old boy named Lee, who had been diagnosed as autistic at age three by Dr. Kanner, was referred to her for treatment. At that point, she knew nothing about autism. Now school aged, Lee was severely self-injurious and aggressive. (Jeanne describes her outpatient success with him in chapter 11 of this book.) Remarkably, she arranged for Lee's removal from institutional care and placement in her own home for intensive treatment. Realizing that she knew "next to nothing about children like Lee," she urgently sought advice from Dr. Kanner, then director of child psychiatry at Johns Hopkins, hoping for his blessing and to benefit from his expertise. Hearing her plan, she said, Dr. Kanner looked at her in disbelief, and then, finally, he spoke: "It's worth a try."

Jeanne was greatly relieved. Thus began their remarkable lifetime collaboration.

Linwood Children's Center in Ellicott City, Maryland, was founded by Jeanne several years later, in 1955, initially enrolling ten children. Dr. Kanner pledged his full support and was delighted when Linwood flourished. He recognized and applauded the dedication, empathy, patience, and idealism that Jeanne blended into a realistic treatment approach. Buoyed by his support, Jeanne pioneered autism treatment at Linwood that over the years garnered international acclaim. Years later, Dr. Kanner published a clinical report attesting to the success of Jeanne's innovative method of treatment.

I first met Jeanne Simons in the 1970s during my fellowship training in child psychiatry. The experience of working with a child diagnosed as autistic had convinced me to pursue a fellowship in child psychiatry after completing my pediatric training at Johns Hopkins. Dr. Kanner was still active as emeritus professor in those years, and I learned about autism diagnosis from him. His first descriptions of autism in 1943 and 1944 included children whose behavior defied traditional psychiatric labels. His first publications were collaborative accounts that incorporated parents' descriptions of their children.

I knew Jeanne as the leader of the Linwood Center, where she pioneered methods of reaching out empathetically to teach children on the autism spectrum. I learned from her how to engage affected children and what mattered in their treatment, but I never thought or suspected that she viewed herself as being on the autism spectrum until I read her life story. Jeanne always insisted her interventions with children were not intuitive but were based on her careful observations.

We now learn for the first time that these observations were informed by her sensitive, subjective self-observations that enhanced her empathy, understanding, and patience with the children she served. Jeanne's success in so effectively engaging these children was informed by her own self-diagnosis of autism spectrum disorder. Reflecting on her early life, she describes how, as a child, she cognitively retreated behind a metaphorical one-way observational mirror, cognitively suppressed her panic when overwhelmed by emotional relationships, and followed self-imposed obsessive rituals to maintain emotional stability—all of which fit into what we now classify as a broad autism spectrum diagnosis. Jeanne did not recognize that she was autistic herself until sometime in the early 1960s, by which point Linwood had already become internationally known. It was a joking comment by a visitor that her uncanny ability to access these children almost suggested that she had had similar experiences that shocked her into realizing that this was indeed true. Jeanne tells us that when her siblings visited Linwood from The Netherlands in later years, they marveled at how similar Jeanne was in her own childhood to the children diagnosed with autism.

Jeanne's self-diagnosis of autism spectrum disorder remains unique among reports by others diagnosed with autism who have written their life histories. Learning about her experience helps me better understand her capacity to engage children with autism. Jeanne tells us in chapter 10 that in the early 1950s she met her first high-functioning adults who were autistic. They were the parents of a child referred to her for treatment. Without being able to conceptualize when she met them how exactly they differed from the norm, she realized only retrospectively that she had something in common with them in her difficulties dealing with emotions. Dr. Kanner recognized autistic traits in parents, too, in his first publication, finding that many were highly accomplished but perfectionistic and interpersonally emotionally distant. Later he described such parents as "successfully autistic." We would now refer to these parents as being "on the autism spectrum."

To fully appreciate Jeanne's self-description as autistic, we must keep in mind that most of the literature on high-functioning people with an autism spectrum diagnosis focuses on men. There is far less written about high-functioning women. High-functioning girls are reported better able to control their emotions outside the home and in school and are better at using gestures and carrying on a conversation. At home, they tend to be prone to anxiety and "emotional meltdowns" like those Jeanne learned to control. Teachers more often focus on boys, whose behavior tends to be more disruptive. Still, both sexes on the autism spectrum have difficulty understanding social relationships.

Mary Temple Grandin is one of the best-known high-functioning adult spokespersons with an autism diagnosis. She is a professor of animal science and consultant to the livestock industry on animal behavior. In her book *Emergence: Labeled Autistic,* she writes from the perspective of her autism diagnosis (2). Grandin has devoted herself to animal welfare, and she has changed practices in animal care to make them more humane. Yet as a child she was labeled as different and was teased and bullied. In contrast, Jeanne tells us that she was not recognized as so clearly different in childhood. Instead, she was acknowledged by her family for her determination and sense of responsibility. As a child, Jeanne apparently successfully sought not to draw attention to herself.

The year I was introduced to Jeanne, I began a combined program in child psychiatry and neurodevelopmental disabilities at what is now the Johns Hopkins Kennedy Krieger Institute. Every week I organized a psychiatry conference for faculty and staff. One of the first people I invited to speak was Jeanne Simons. I asked her to illustrate how she engaged an child who had autism. Even today I vividly remember the video she showed us. The child with autism who was shown in the video hid under a blanket and was revealed and engaged by Jeanne through a game of peek-a-boo. In the early 1980s, I founded the Johns Hopkins autism clinic at the Kennedy Institute with Dennis Whitehouse and pursued what I had learned from Jeanne in autism assessment and treatment.

Jeanne's early education as a preschool teacher with additional training as a Montessori teacher prepared her for her later work with children with autism. Maria Montessori began her career working with children with mental disabilities, especially intellectual disability. Montessori focused on children becoming independent as an aim of education, with the role of the teacher being an observer who facilitated children's self-motivated psychological development. Through her philosophy of following the child's lead, Jeanne adapted this philosophy in her work with children who were diagnosed as autistic. Thus, Jeanne emphasized that we begin by watching where the child is focusing his attention and then follow his lead, slowly nudging him toward social interactions. If a young child with autism loves to spin, one might use the spinning to make contact with him by picking the child up and spinning with him in a circle until he makes eye contact, then putting the child down. When he wants to spin again, one might require him to hold out both arms to signal wanting to be picked up to spin, thus shaping a socially appropriate behavior.

I stayed in touch with Jeanne and Linwood through their thirtieth, fortieth, and fiftieth anniversaries and was a speaker at the thirtieth and fortieth anniversaries. I continue to treat adults in the Linwood autism adult residential program whom I have followed for more than twenty-five years. The work Jeanne started continues there, and her sensitive developmental approach, informed by behavioral analysis, focused on socially engaging children with autism, is now widely emulated. Her emphasis on affective engagement and intersubjectivity is incorporated in autism treatment programs in many US schools—for example, the Early Start Denver Model. This method has been shown effective in randomized, double-blind, controlled treatment studies. And Jeanne's treatment philosophy lives on in the new Linwood School Program in a larger, more modern facility. In its new incarnation it is certified as a treatment program by the state of Maryland.

In summary, I found Jeanne's life story as detailed in this book to be riveting, as I learned how she mastered her own autistic inner turmoil and social perplexity. She movingly explains how these personal life experiences and choices led to her finding a way to engage children who were once thought lost and not engageable. Thank you, Jeanne!

James C. Harris, MD

Founding Director, Developmental Neuropsychiatry
Professor of Psychiatry and Behavioral Sciences,
Mental Health, Pediatrics, and History of Medicine
The Johns Hopkins University School of Medicine
and Bloomberg School of Public Health

REFERENCES

1. Simons, J., & Oishi, S. The Hidden Child: The Linwood Method for Reaching the Autistic Child. Baltimore, MD: Woodbine House, 1987.
2. Grandin, T., & Scariano, M. M. Emergence: Labeled Autistic. New York: Grand Central Publishing, 1996 (1986).

Preface

I first met Jeanne Simons in 1983, a few years after she had retired as director of the Linwood Children's Center, a treatment facility for children and adolescents living with autism, which she had founded. For almost three decades she had trained staff and visiting professionals by example, but as she was handing off the running of Linwood to others, people in the autism community around her were increasingly concerned about the need to codify her method and write it down while she was still in good health, and they were looking for someone to help with this task. Such a guide would benefit parents and anyone else living and working with children with seemingly intractable emotional and behavioral problems, like the ones who had motivated her to start her center.

I had long been interested in autism and the work done at Linwood. So, after completing a doctorate in human development at the University of Maryland, I jumped at the opportunity to help sift through and organize existing material, flesh it out by personal observations and ongoing conversations with Jeanne Simons, and come up with a description of the treatment methods she had developed.

As it turned out, Jeanne and I were a good match, and over the course of an intensive year's work the project matured into the book *The Hidden Child*, published in 1987 by Woodbine House (1). In the process of working together on the book, we also became friends—a friendship that deepened over time and immeasurably enriched my life until Jeanne's death in 2005.

When I started my work, I had no inkling that Jeanne herself was autistic, though it had struck me as unusual that when she recounted case histories from her earliest years as a therapist, they did not differ in the telling by so much as a single word from audio recorded or written-down versions of the same case histories I found in the materials accumulated over decades that I was working through. Even people with a photographic memory tend to leave out something, add some detail, or use different words when they describe a past incident, but Jeanne's stories never varied. It was as if she was reading from an inner monitor to describe a scene unfolding in the present. Many of these case histories also revealed her uncanny ability to tap into a child's behavior in the exact right way and at the exact time when it could be changed. But she became upset whenever someone attributed this ability to "intuition." She insisted with some vehemence that it was really only close and patient observation that dictated the correct timing of an intervention, and that anybody with the appropriate training and patience could do what she did.

Then one day she handed me a few typewritten pages, yellow with age. As I discovered, they were not another case study, like the previous materials I had gone through, but a vignette from her own early childhood. The account was vividly written. It also unmistakably revealed the child in the story as being an individual with autism. I was stunned and confused. Had she given me this memoir with the intention of telling me something, albeit indirectly? Or did she not realize what she was describing?

But this was Jeanne Simons. I could not imagine that this pioneer in the treatment of autism would not have recognized the behavior and reactions of her younger self as those typical of such a child. When I finally diffidently asked my question, I discovered that Jeanne had indeed known for decades about her autism. She made no secret about her condition but also saw no need to broadcast it, any more than she would have any other personal information. Yet she clearly wanted me to know, and I felt honored by her trust.

She later talked to me about the sense of relief this self-discovery had afforded her, because she could finally make sense of the differences she had observed between the way she reacted to her surroundings, people, and events and the behavior of others. Early on she had developed strategies that helped her successfully navigate the minefield of her condition. In fact, she never did see it as a disability but accepted it as the blueprint and determinant for her life's work. But she was eventually able to admit that her affinity with these youngsters was at least partly due to her recognizing something in them that mirrored her own experience.

Jeanne and I had many long conversations about her life, and the more she told me about herself the clearer it became to me that this was a story that needed to be published, because her experiences provided an amazing window into the mind and sensibility of someone on the autism spectrum, albeit someone of uncommon intellect, functioning at the high end of the spectrum. After initial reticence, Jeanne became increasingly enthusiastic about the idea of writing down and publishing her life story.

Even before *The Hidden Child* was published, I was spending whatever free time I had listening to and recording her tales, sorting through the recollections she had written down, and asking questions to close gaps in the narrative.

The original manuscript for Jeanne's life story was finished in 1989. Once Jeanne was satisfied with it we started thinking of ways to get it published. I sent the manuscript off to an agent who, recognizing the importance of the work to the field of autism, expressed great enthusiasm for it. When he had not been able to find us a publisher by 1992, however, it became clear that we might have to rethink our approach.

Feedback from select friends and professionals indicated a need to restructure and annotate the text in ways that would make it more comprehensible to readers who had no expertise in the field of autism and who could not be expected to fully appreciate the importance of what Jeanne related in her memoir.

Pressure of work and other life events intervened, and the manuscript remained in the drawer. But even as Jeanne's health began to decline and her short-term memory deteriorated, she often remembered additional episodes that she thought were of interest and needed to be included.

We had not talked about the book project as such for a number of years when, at what turned out to be our last visit, in 2005, Jeanne said, "I have been thinking about something all of last week that I wanted to ask you about. What is happening with our book?" I told her that I had not yet found a publisher. We had never bothered to draw up a formal agreement, but she had always told me that she wanted me to have sole rights to her story, and we had agreed that I would share any profits from this project with Linwood. She reiterated her wish that I pursue publication, but she also wanted to make sure that I had included her earliest memory, which she described to me again in minute detail.

Jeanne died barely two weeks after this conversation, but her request gave me the push I needed to pick up where we had left off and to start reworking the manuscript in a way that I hoped would make the life and mind of this remarkable woman accessible to a wide readership. *Behind the Mirror* is my attempt to keep this promise.

Jeanne's own writing and the way she told her story to me is vivid and evocative. I was careful not to tamper with the recollections she had written down herself, other than to address grammatical idiosyncrasies that were due her being born in Belgium and raised in Holland. English was an adopted language.

While I kept scrupulously to the facts as Jeanne presented them, it is inevitable that in transcribing conversations that went on over days and months, my own voice intrudes. But in *Behind the Mirror*, as in *The Hidden Child*, Jeanne carefully read and if necessary edited and corrected everything I had written, which also gave her an opportunity to further develop a theme.

In reworking the book, I eventually trimmed down Jeanne's memoir to those parts that touched directly on her own challenges as well as on her teaching methods, because while her whole life story is a riveting read, it is those parts that set this account apart from any other written about living with autism. The finished project is an annotated memoir as told to me, because Jeanne's voice is so extraordinary and important that I did not want to lose it by turning the book into a biography—all the more so as there were things that despite my training I never really "got," especially the absolutely vital importance of some of the coping mechanisms she developed to be able to function. (I include one example of my not "getting it" in chapter 2.)

There were other differences between us that stemmed from Jeanne's ASD that we could nail down but understand only intellectually. One of these was the different way we functioned as therapists and teachers. Let me say here that in the context of working with children with autism, the roles of therapist and teacher are interchangeable, because all educational work with these children requires a therapeutic approach.

Typical therapists, as well as teachers, not only invest a lot of energy, thought, and caring in their clients, but over time develop a therapeutic relationship with them within which the magic of healing and learning takes place. But, as is discussed later in this book, individuals living with autism tend not to develop deep emotional bonds, so the relationship between them and their teachers stays emotionally one-sided. This can make working with children with ASD draining—unless the teacher lacks the need for such a bond, as well, as was true for Jeanne. Understanding that she was an exception, Jeanne stressed that anyone working with such individuals must have a rich and satisfying emotional life outside their professional activities, to make up for the slow progress they make and the dearth of emotional feedback they provide.

I need to add that many of the terms Jeanne used, such as *handicapped* rather than *disabled* or *an autistic child* rather than *a child with ASD*, reflect an outdated vocabulary that may be offensive to a modern reader. But they are authentic to the era when she worked with children with autism and to her voice, and it would have been anachronistic to replace them with modern usage. I have, however, taken care to upgrade my own vocabulary around the topic, which has been a challenge, since even people within the autism community cannot always agree on terms.

It is also important to state that this book was never conceived as a "how to" guide for parents and educators, though some autism resources are listed in appendix B. There are many excellent such books on the market as well as moving testimonies of teachers and parents of what working and living with a child on the spectrum is like (2).

To say that Jeanne Simons' life with autism was unique is to ignore that the experiences, predominant challenges, and the life trajectory of every individual, including those on the spectrum, are unique. As will quickly become apparent to readers, Jeanne exhibited a significant number of symptoms attributable to ASD, though she functioned at the high end of the spectrum. There are, however, some very unusual characteristics that make her stand out.

Remarkably, she was able, from her earliest, possibly preverbal, childhood, to analyze the challenges posed by her symptoms and adjust her behavior in ways that kept her from being noticed. It apparently was accepted in her family that she was somehow different, but since she never posed a problem and was successful in school, no one seemed to have thought much about this difference. She was, in fact, hiding in full sight all of her life.

Another difference is that while there are many individuals with autism who end up leading independent and successful lives, they mostly tend toward fields that require relatively little interaction with or dependence on others, with careers that are based on logical thinking, like mathematics or IT or the physical sciences, or possibly as writers, rather than in fields that require a lot of verbal interactions or human relations.

In contrast, Jeanne knew from the time she was a young child that her vocation was to work with children who needed help. Her choice of education and every job she ever had reflected her calling. Though she felt that her ability to form deep and lasting relationships was deficient, her own autism informed work that required children to become comfortable and trusting in a relationship with her or other teachers. Her empathy with struggling parents and her ability to "read" others eventually led to her pioneering treatment approach with children with ASD that helped so many of them emerge from the confines their condition imposed.

And lastly, individuals on the spectrum are often nonverbal or are unable to access, understand, manage, or succinctly talk about their experiences. There are therefore few accounts of how a person with an ASD diagnosis experiences the world, the most famous exception being Temple Grandin (3, 4). Some fascinating first-person accounts by young authors from across the world (5, 6, 7), also fall in this category. They will be made more accessible to readers who have been guided through this complex terrain by a person like Jeanne Simons, who not only had uncommon insight into her condition but was able to describe it in vivid detail.

Her account should leave readers with a clearer understanding of why children with autism act the way they do, including why they may react so strongly and at times disconcertingly to seemingly innocuous stimuli or situations. This understanding will, I hope, also help caregivers see these behaviors for what they are: the children's reactions to the confusing, frightening, or even painful experience they have to deal with and defend against day in and day out. Rather than rejecting actions as "bad," it encourages caregivers to look for and encourage their charges' strengths, thus creating an optimal environment for them.

For the general public, Jeanne's story may help demystify the subject of autism, situating it among the many disabilities with which the differently abled can, with early intervention, the proper support, and societal acceptance, share in the pursuit of happiness that is the birthright of every child. It is ultimately a story about possibilities and hope.

REFERENCES

1. Simons, J., & Oishi, S. The Hidden Child: The Linwood Method for Reaching the Autistic Child. Baltimore, MD: Woodbine House, 1987.
2. Bucher, R. D. A Mommy, a Daddy, Two Sisters, and a Jimmy: Autism and the Difference It Makes. Self-published 2019. rdbucher@aol.com
3. Grandin, T., & Scariano, M. M. Emergence: Labeled Autistic. New York: Grand Central Publishing, 1996 (1986).
4. Grandin, T. Thinking in Pictures: My Life with Autism. New York: Doubleday, 1995.
5. Higashida, N. The Reason I Jump. New York: Random House, 2013 (first published in Japanese by Escor Publishers, 2007).
6. Robison, J. E. Look Me in the Eye: My Life with Asperger's. New York: Broadway Books, 2007.
7. Williams, D. Nobody, Nowhere: The Remarkable Autobiography of an Autistic Girl. New York: Avon Books, 1992.

Behind the mirror

Introduction
A brief description of early autism development

What he called *infantile autism* was first described in 1943 by Dr. Leo Kanner as a neurodevelopmental disorder present from the beginning of life. It is now formally known as autism spectrum disorder (ASD) to indicate the full range of severity, including intellectual functioning and behavioral manifestations, grouped within this one diagnostic category.

The possible causes of this disorder are yet to be determined. Genetic, neuropsychological, neurobiological, and environmental factors have been identified, but the ultimate answers remain elusive. An account of the latest state of research into the etiology of ASD is presented by Dr. James C. Harris in appendix A.

Over the past seventy-six years, both professionals and the general public have become more aware of the existence of ASD, in good part because its prevalence has increased to the point where it could almost be termed a mental health epidemic. (Dr. Harris addresses some possible reasons for this phenomenon in appendix A as well.) What has not changed is that a diagnosis of autism is based strictly on observable behavioral symptoms in various categories, like cognitive and social skills development and language, as well as on abnormal behavioral manifestations, such as compulsions or oversensitivity to sensory input. The latest description of these behavioral symptoms and abnormal behavioral manifestations that lead to an ASD diagnosis are encrypted in the diagnostic and statistical manuals issued and edited periodically by the American Psychiatric Association (for details, see appendix A).

Concerns have been raised that by now ASD has become so "popularized" that it is often diagnosed or treated by people not qualified to do so. It has been, and remains, one of the most difficult disorders to properly diagnose and treat, yet the earlier a formal diagnosis is made by a trained professional and appropriate medication treatment and education are started, the greater is the likelihood of recovery, which in the context of this disorder means the ability to function in the community and ideally in a regular school or work environment, and to live independently.

Treatment approaches have also evolved over time. In the epilogue I describe the Linwood method developed by Jeanne Simons and some of what today are known as "best practices."

TO ORIENT THE READER to the child and adult they will encounter in Jeanne Simons' account in the following pages, this introduction briefly outlines normal child development and describes observable ways development and behaviors take different paths in a child with autism. I will be using the pronoun *he* throughout, since autism occurs four times more often among boys than girls. As in any description of human development, including those of children with any type of disability, there is a wide range in both the timing and the quality of developmental steps. There is always a lower/slower end and a faster/higher end of what is described as the norm, with few children falling cleanly into the "average" middle in every aspect of their development or abilities.

Imagine a normal—what is now often referred to as *neurotypical*—newborn. His needs are few and basic. He cries when he is hungry, maybe when he is colicky or wet. Picked up, changed, fed, and cuddled, he quiets immediately. Within days, he will open his eyes and look up into the face of his mother while he nurses. It is a steady, clear-eyed gaze, as if he is intently memorizing every feature. Mother and child, wrapped up in each other, gazing at each other, reestablish the connection disrupted by the trauma of birth. The bond they forge through the hours, days, and weeks of caregiving will not only be the strongest and most enduring of all human bonds but also provide the template for all future relationships.

Tenderly, the mother looks down at her baby. She smiles at him, and one day, eagerly awaited and a miracle every time, the baby smiles back. He does not smile at his bottle or the mobile above his bed or at pictures. He only smiles at the sight of the human face, the first indication that, in just six short weeks of life, he has learned to distinguish objects from people. This is a social smile, the first sign of active participation in reciprocal, social interactions.

Vocalizing increases as caregivers coo back at him. The baby picks up pitch and variations in tone. He can reproduce a melodic line before he is one year old. Meaning gets attached to syllables. Activities become purposeful. In the give and take of play, the child becomes increasingly aware of himself and others as different individuals. By age three, he will talk about himself in the first person.

When he hurts himself, he cries. He looks to the caregivers for solace, succor, and approval, clapping his hands when he has achieved a difficult feat. Their encouragement feeds his determination. In play, the baby explores his world. Every aspect of a new object is examined. He tastes, smells, pokes, bangs, studies his toys. In a few brief months, play becomes imitation. He vacuums busily with a piece of hose. He wipes and stirs. By age three, imitation segues into make-believe. He pretends to be a kitten or a lion. A blanket over a chair becomes a house.

Imagination and reality now become separate realms in which he moves at will, although his understanding of the world is still wholly informed by how things appear, what can be observed and experienced. The moon still follows him around. He is convinced that there is more water in a tall thin glass than in a squat wide one, even though he has seen the same amount poured into each, because the water level in one is visibly higher than in the other. He thinks in concrete terms and takes things literally.

But by the time he is ready to go to school, he will have learned to think about things from different points of view. Basic reasoning emerges, based on the ability to deduce and to generalize. Two plus two make four—always. He loves nonsense words, rhymes, and word games. He delights in slapstick and surprises. Humor, the ability to enjoy the absurd, is the flip side of being able to abstract. The ability for formal, logical thinking is but a step away.

YOU WILL NOT MEET such a child in the following account of Jeanne Simons' life. This baby, this child, and those who, like her, are born with autism spectrum disorder, differ in most important aspects from the development described above. Sometimes these differences are subtle and a diagnosis is difficult before age three or four; sometimes they are striking. Let me highlight a number of them for you, so you will recognize them more easily when you encounter them in the following memoir or in real life.

A baby with autism cannot be comforted. He shrinks from the tender touch and the sound of the loving voice of his caretakers. He stiffens when he is picked up, arches away from contact, turns his head. His gaze does not engage. He looks past and through his mother. There is no social smile, no interchange of cooing, no gesturing for attention, no acknowledgment that people are different from bottles or pictures. He treats people like other objects in his environment. He may even try to use them like tools, their hand or arm an extension of his, a stick to reach for something he wants.

This child does not look to his caretakers for comfort when he hurts himself. In fact, he often does not seem to register that he is hurt, or at least he does not visibly react. It almost seems that he does not realize that the toe he stubbed, the head he bumped, belongs to him. On the other hand, these children may be hypersensitive to all kinds of sensations. They may flinch from light or sound, may not tolerate certain tactile sensations, or may overreact to smells. They might eat dirt or leaves but refuse most regular foods or have distinct and narrow food preferences.

A child with autism seems oblivious to praise or approval. He may be mute or repeat words or even whole phrases verbatim, but not as part of a game, or in order to communicate, but mechanically or compulsively. Some children may exhibit an unusual ability to remember and reproduce a melody, but they do not sing along with others. More often such a child hums tunelessly to himself as he goes through repetitive motions, isolated in a world of his own. He may appear deaf, because he often does not react even to loud noises. Oblivious to his surroundings he flaps his fingers, twirls objects, spins the wheels on toy cars and trucks, or rocks back and forth. These stereotyped movements seem to have an almost hypnotic effect on the child. But even as they soothe him, they further insulate and thus isolate him from the outside world.

This child is not spontaneous. He is not eager to expand his world and explore new things. Instead, he tends to compulsively arrange random objects, food, toys, and (later) books and even furniture in rigid patterns. If these arrangements are disturbed, or if there are any other changes in his environment or his routine, he becomes inordinately distressed and agitated. At those times, or even without a visible trigger, he may go into violent temper tantrums.

There is no imitative play that grooms him for his later roles in life. There is no make-believe. This child is yoked to his immediate experiences. He remains, throughout life, a concrete thinker, taking everything literally. In *The Hidden Child*, the book I coauthored with Jeanne, we give a number of examples of this literalness (1). One youngster was instructed to "draw the woods" after coming back from a walk. He drew a number of sticks—which, for him, was the plural of "wood." You will find many striking examples of this concrete thinking and literalness in the following pages.

The child with autism does not seem to delight in the company of others. If he plays at all, it is in isolation. If others get in his way, he walks around them or pushes them aside as if they were pieces of furniture. This inability to relate is at the heart of autism. It is its most striking characteristic and the most serious handicap. The lack of human connectedness has tellingly been called "autistic aloneness." It is the hardest symptom to diagnose and the hardest to treat. Whether immediately discernible or largely hidden, it is present even in highly intelligent individuals with autism, whose cognitive and language development may be minimally impaired. It shapes the child and sets him apart throughout life in ways that are so foreign to the experience of others that it is extremely difficult to find words to describe them. Some authors posit that emotional poverty and an aversion to company are not symptoms of autism but consequences of it, the product of the "harsh lockdown on self-expression and society's near-pristine ignorance of what's happening inside autistic heads" (2). But the fact remains that emotions are so difficult for individuals with autism that even those who can converse appropriately and freely on factual topics may revert to mutism or monosyllabic answers when asked about issues with any kind of emotional overtone.

REFERENCES

1. Simons, J., & Oishi, S. The Hidden Child: The Linwood Method for Reaching the Autistic Child. Baltimore, MD: Woodbine House, 1987.
2. Williams, D. Nobody, Nowhere: The Remarkable Autobiography of an Autistic Girl. New York: Avon Books, 1992.

Birth, 1909

I was told much later that mine had been a difficult birth. When I was finally born, my mother's life hung in the balance. Neither doctor nor midwife had a thought to spare for the little girl who had been born with the cord wrapped around her neck and with the fetal membrane covering her head. Under it, I was described as having been a dusky blue. They labored over my mother until the worst of the hemorrhaging stopped. She was young and strong. God willing, she would recover.

My mother slept, too weak to ask after her child, who had lain there, not crying, unattended, and given up for dead. But when the midwife lifted up the little body, the baby was still breathing. It was days before my skin took on a more normal hue. When after four days my mother was judged strong enough to see me for the first time, I was still faintly mauve, and instead of turning eagerly to the comforting breast, I pushed at it with tightly curled fists, turning my head and crying in protest. I would go rigid when I was held, and respond to attempts to soothe me by scrunching up my eyes and tensing my whole body. I could not be breastfed but accepted a bottle. But I seemed to be healthy, despite my inauspicious beginnings and the constant wailing that seemed to signal some terrible pain.

All of this Jeanne had been told, but as incredible as it may sound, the adult claims to remember this pain more than eighty years later. As she struggles to talk about it, she seems to relive it. Her body tenses.

The language she is forced to invent to convey this earliest of memories frustrates her. Her hands flutter and her face tightens. How to describe sensations before there are words, sensations that are indescribable with even the most sophisticated vocabulary?

She remembers how the sound of her mother's voice sent something resembling a thousand little electrical impulses through her body. Such torture can never be forgotten. The mother's voice is soft, full of emotion. It pierces the baby. The breast, too soft, too close, suffocates. The baby fights for breath, she fights for survival. The whole period of her early life is a desperate struggle to keep herself intact, to shut out sights, sounds, feelings that threaten to blow her apart. The newborn has few defenses. Only screaming to ward off intolerable intrusions and to block out the pain.

Oral traditions attribute to children born with a caul that they are destined to lead a charmed life, that they can see into the future and that everything they do turns out well for them. In German, the caul is called *die Glückshaut*—the skin that brings luck. This child would need all the luck she could get. What follows is the story of this child and of the challenges, as well as the gifts, she was born with.

Early memories

2

I was born in Belgium, the country of my mother, in December of 1909. Behind our house there was a garden. My mother was an avid gardener and grew beautiful roses. As babies we were wheeled out into the garden, with a light veil thrown over the carriage to protect us against insects.

My earliest memory is of lying in the basket with a soft, shimmering light over me. I also remember the smell of the roses wafting over me. There is a sense of peacefulness, of nothingness. Then everything changes. Suddenly there is nothing but pain. It is like being blown into a thousand small pieces. There is pain without hurt, and then there is terror without knowing what terror is. The little pieces scramble together again, whirling into a ball, only to be blown apart again, and then try and try and finally get together again. Then the peace and nothingness return.

Roses bloom early in Belgium, so it was probably May, and I was perhaps five months old at the time of this memory. I think that the pain that threatened to explode my fragile self, awash in light and the scent of roses, came from the intrusion of my mother's voice. My mother had a beautiful voice and she loved babies. When she spoke to them, her voice was soft and gentle.

Yet to me, it was almost unbearably painful. I do not know why. But I knew instinctively that unless I could block it out, it might destroy me. Even today, when I smell a rose or see light shine through a veil, it can make me feel incredibly peaceful. And it can make me lose all sense of time and shift me way back, where I am drifting weight-lessly in warmth and light. The peacefulness is seductive and danger-ous. It would be so easy to stay there forever. For that reason, I avoid roses and am afraid of them, while at the same time they attract me.

I cried from the time I was a little baby. I cried especially hard when we went somewhere. I think my mother thought that I cried because she wasn't there. But that wasn't true at all. What terrified me was the change. I was taken from an environment I knew and where I felt relatively safe to one that was unfamiliar, and therefore unpre-dictable and threatening. How could I protect myself against painful experiences when I didn't know what to anticipate? Even familiar people became strangers to me in a new environment, so I couldn't rely on them to act in known ways.

All my life transitions have been very difficult for me. But as a small child without an understanding of what was to come, the "in-between" times were especially scary. I remember once when my mother was ready to take me out, she set me down on the floor for a moment. I was all dressed up in a little lacy bonnet. I could see the light through its brim and can still feel the terror of sitting on the floor, faced with the unknown. Then my hand touched the tiles. There were grooves in them. They had a pattern to them, which I could follow with my fin-ger. I traced the lines over and over again. The terror receded. I did not feel anything anymore. But for years a hat on a baby's head both-ered me. I always tried to take it off, because a hat means that you are going somewhere and you are taken from an environment that is fa-miliar and safe.

When I was still little enough to be picked up, we often went to visit my grandparents who lived a few hours from Brussels. My mother came too, but I cried inconsolably. I did not know where I was. In the strange environment, my mother was different. My grand-parents, who must have visited us in Brussels, were different. My aunts seemed strangers.

When I cried and protested, everyone tried to comfort me by pick-ing me up, but I hated being touched and this only made me cry harder.

Then one day I suddenly made the connection between my crying and being picked up. I still remember that moment of understanding and the conclusion I drew from it. I decided that I should not cry anymore. This was terribly difficult, because crying had been an outlet for my pain, but from that moment on the crying stopped and I do not remember being picked up anymore.

Sometime after that I had a bad earache. It hurt so much it made me cry, and of course I got taken care of. I remember feeling helpless because I couldn't stop crying and drawing so much attention to myself. The intensity of my mother and my aunt hovering over me was very painful, and from then on I tried to keep any discomfort or illness to myself. I succeeded so well that on one occasion I almost died, but I did not cry again for over twenty years.

For a time, the crying was replaced by stiffening the whole body when something frightening happened. I had done this ever since I was a baby, but now I would stiffen my body for a long time and even hold my breath for a while. When I did this I felt protected, as if I were in a glass bubble. I could look out but nobody could look in, and I could not feel their touch. By and by I learned to make myself blind and deaf against anything that might hurt me, especially emotions. I also developed ways to distract myself from emotions that crowded in on me by focusing on something else: the hypnotic rhythm of repetitive movements, like rocking, or the sensation of a texture, a pattern of lines or colors.

I was fifteen months old when my first brother was born. I was carried to a neighbor's house where my sister and I sat on a wooden floor. I remember the beginnings of something like panic at this sudden and inexplicable change. I can still remember the glossy paper and the musty smell of old books. I am holding this huge book, the size of an atlas, on my lap. It had pictures in it. They were black and white. The pages were thick and bulged a little in the middle. I put my hands on the book and moved them over the smooth pages, back and forth, back and forth, savoring the feel of the paper and the special smell of the book. I was totally consumed by these sensations, and the panic subsided.

As I got older I became better at distracting myself. The sight of familiar objects was reassuring and I selected them to focus on, such as the buttons on my shoes or the glints of light reflecting off the polished brass trimming of the stove. And during a period of frequent moves, I carried a little piece of flowered wallpaper from our old house around with me. I touched it and looked at it. Or I touched some lace on my dress, or a ribbon. They made a soft sound, a sound I could feel rather than hear. It always brought the great, quiet emptiness I needed and moved the world away from me.

There was no way that I could understand then just what it was that frightened me to the point of disintegration. But the older I grew the better I became at finding practical solutions to protect myself from sudden changes or things I could not understand that could have made me anxious enough to threaten me in some way.

When my next brother, Dominique, was born, I was two and a half years old. As was customary, my mother had the baby at home. It may have been simply the heightened emotions in the house or the commotion and change of routine that threw me off course. In any case, I went absolutely rigid and for the longest time I refused to eat or drink anything. The doctor was the only one who sensed that something was very wrong. I remember standing outside my mother's bedroom door. It had a transom through which I could hear them talking. Later, my mother told me that she had been worried about something to do with the baby, and that the doctor had told her that she should worry more about me than about the new baby. But no one took him seriously.

An aunt had come to look after us while my mother was recovering. My sister, who was two years older than I, asked her why my mother was sick. In explanation, our aunt told us the following story: "Once in a while, people receive a postcard. It tells the mother to come to a certain place where there are barges full of babies. On these ships are sailors from Spain or maybe Africa. They are black. The mother has to come by herself, and while she picks up the baby, these people beat her and she has to run very fast to try and get away so she won't get hurt too badly. Sometimes she is in luck and can get a carriage, and then she escapes without much damage."

Naturally I believed this scary story in its entirety. To deal with the fears it raised, I had to do something. I figured that if there was no postcard, there was no need to go to the barge. I could protect my mother from getting hurt by destroying the postcard. Our mail was delivered through a slot in the front door. For days I watched the mailbox, until one day there was a postcard among the mail. I have no memory of ripping it up, but I must have done so, because from that day on I was at ease. The whole topic was completely off my mind. Even though my mother had three more children, I never again worried about it. I did better than that. I managed not to notice that she was pregnant at all, even though I was seventeen when my youngest sister was born.

But at one point or another it must have been explained to me that babies come out of the womb. I don't remember exactly when the realization came to me that this might have been true for my own birth as well. Before the feelings of unbearable closeness to the mother and the sense of suffocation that this thought evoked could overwhelm me, I focused on a tree I happened to be looking at. A tree is something stable and predictable. It is always there. It is hard. You can hold on to it and it doesn't smother you. It doesn't answer back. It doesn't move away. Even though I knew better, from that time on, I thought of myself as having been born from a tree. This thought defended me against an unacceptable reality.

The older I got the easier it became to anticipate difficult situations and to protect myself against them. But when I was little, I was still very vulnerable and was often taken by surprise. I remember, for example, the experience that led to my unease with presents.

We were still living in Belgium and I was perhaps four or five years old. Our neighbor had a big old lilac tree. I remember a man, standing on a ladder, cutting lilacs. I was outside, watching him, and he climbed down and filled my little apron with them. I remember the starched pleats of the apron, the pure joy of holding the fragrant branches in it, and the perfume that enveloped me. I carried them indoors and then, suddenly, they were gone. Someone must have taken them from me to put them in a vase. But to me, it was the abrupt end to a wonderful feeling. It was something I had to close off from. It was too painful to feel this bliss and then to lose it. After that, I never trusted presents again, because they might turn out to harbor some hurt.

When Jeanne told me this story, my heart hurt for the little girl whose loss of the beautiful lilacs was so huge that it spoiled her pleasure in all future gifts.

At some later time, the lilacs in my garden produced an unusually large and beautiful crop. I was going to visit Jeanne, so I cut a big armful of lilacs to bring to her, hoping to make up for her early pain and perhaps restore to her what she had lost.

I cannot now remember how she received my gift. She must have put the flowers in water, and if she reacted, it cannot have been in any way that alerted me that there was anything wrong. But years later, when we had become close enough friends so she felt safe with me, Jeanne finally reacted to my present. We were discussing how hard it was for an outsider to understand the emotional makeup and needs of autistic individuals. Suddenly she said quietly, "You know, even you don't really understand. Remember when you brought me that lilac. You almost killed me."

I must have gaped at her aghast. "I told you how I had to close myself off from that hurt so it would not destroy me," she said. "Then you brought me the flowers, and their scent brought it all back and threatened to break through my protection. I wasn't sure whether I was going to be able to keep myself from fragmenting and to close it all off again."

It was not until then that I got an inkling of how dangerous emotions can be to individuals with autism. Jeanne herself could never explain why this should be so. I also appreciated fully for the first time the minefield one has to negotiate when dealing with an autistic individual. It was a powerful experience and a lesson in humility to realize that unwittingly I had come so close to harming someone I loved and admired.

At around the same time, I also lost the ability to be afraid. We lived in a house with a cellar that was dark and cool and where food was stored. My sister was supposed to fetch something from the cellar, but she was afraid to go down there by herself. I sensed her fear and also sensed something in my mother's voice when she asked me to go in my sister's place. I now think that she herself may also have been afraid to go down into the cellar. I needed to protect myself from their feelings, so I quickly agreed to go. It stopped the fear in my mother and my sister, but it also gave me a sense of what fear was, so that I was able to defend against it in myself. From that time on, I have never felt fear in any situation.

What made it harder for me to assess situations was that I took everything completely literally. For that reason, I believed any stories we were told. I did not distinguish between a story and reality. I was very troubled, for example, by a Dutch Christmas song in which Baby Jesus is described as having been blue with cold. I could not understand why Mary would not have wrapped her child in her coat to keep him warm. I was equally unhappy whenever I saw a crèche in which the Christ Child was naked. It puzzled me, and there was no realization that this was just a figure that could not feel anything. To me, there was no difference between objects and people.

I remember once, when we went for a walk, we passed a little open wayside chapel with Jesus on the cross. It was a very cold day and I knew that I had to take off my coat and cover him, since nobody else had thought to do this obvious thing. The adults only saw that I was trying to get out of my coat and wouldn't let me take it off. They never found out what I had in mind, which was just as well, because they might have laughed at me and it would have been hard for me to be the center of attention. I let them lead me away, thinking that I would sneak out at night and go through with my plan, but of course I couldn't, and I blocked it out again.

I could only deal with concrete things. I never had any wishes, because that would have required imagination. It also takes up a lot of energy to want things you may not be able to have. And I also had a very hard time dealing with choices. A choice implies that you change a situation, and since you need imagination to picture what new situation each choice might create, any choice for me meant facing unpredictability. Making choices was in fact so painful that, if possible, I chose not to make any and to just wait. But sometimes that was not possible.

I remember one wartime Christmas when some organization had put on a Christmas party for the children. There was a long table piled with different gifts, and every child was allowed to choose something they wanted. We walked single file along the table, and there were many wonderful things and many things I might have enjoyed, but I did not know what I wanted. I remember someone saying, "Oh look at this" or "Look at that," but I couldn't make a choice. And then we were at the end of the table. So I picked up something at random because it had pretty colors. It turned out to be a little paint set, nothing at all compared to all the other things I had passed up because I couldn't choose.

I still have problems with making choices. It isn't as traumatic anymore, especially if it involves day-to-day decisions. If it is something unimportant, like the choice of a restaurant, for example, I will let the other person make the choice. The big things in my life I have generally just tended to let happen. Except for once, I have never needed to look for a job, for example. They have just come along, and, when they seemed right, there was really no need to make a choice.

Jeanne and I often talked about what might make emotions, their own as well as those of others, so painful and dangerous to many individuals with autism. Jeanne thought that there had to be a neurological explanation. Absent that, as she writes in chapter 13, the closest she could come was to liken herself to someone born without pigmentation. Such people have to avoid the sun at all cost to avoid serious burns. She also hypothesized that the condition might be related in some way to the abnormal reactions to sensory input observed in many autistic individuals, in this case a hypersensitivity to emotional stimuli.

But the need to shut oneself off from emotions is potentially a lot more crippling than an avoidance of direct sunlight, certain foods, or physical sensations. Relationships are based on feelings. Suppressed emotions atrophy the capacity to develop the full gamut of social and emotional interactions. It is something Jeanne struggled with a lot in later life and will be addressed later in the book.

As Jeanne's earliest memories demonstrate, change is especially difficult for children with autism and can even be devastating to them. In a new and strange environment, even familiar people become strangers, because these children experience their environment as a whole, an arrangement within which people are objects among an assembly of other objects.

Childhood during World War I

3

When I was about four and a half, the war started. The Germans immediately invaded Belgium. Within a short time food supplies became scarce and food became more and more expensive. Children from low-income families were fed in the schools, but after a while even children from families that were well off were undernourished. When all the children in my school were examined, it was found that many of them had already developed tuberculosis. About fifty youngsters were still in pretty good shape, and the Red Cross decided to send them to Holland for six weeks, to an environment with plenty of food, so they would have a better chance of coming through the war with their health intact.

The children chosen had to be at least six years old. My sister, who was seven, qualified. I did not, since I was barely five and a half. My parents did not want to send my sister by herself, and they somehow managed to have me included in the group that was to live under the care of Dutch Sisters somewhere at the seashore. All of this must have been explained to me, but if so I did not take it in, because there was too much emotion on the part of my parents. I didn't understand what was going to happen.

All I remember is that I am dressed in a sailor suit. My hair is parted in two braids, with ribbons at the end. The ribbons make a soft sound when I touch them. On my back I have a knapsack with clothes in it. I can feel the pull on my shoulders. There are many children, all dressed alike, with their mothers.

The mothers stand in a line, the children in front of them. It is very dark, and the line is endless. I do not know why we are standing in this dark space. There is crying, and I try not to hear it. I am touching my ribbon. I hear the soft sound. It makes my tears stay in.

Then the soldiers come. They carry rifles with knives at the top. Little lights dance on and off the knives. They are German soldiers. I don't know what that means. There is a sudden silence among the mothers. Now there is only the sound of many footsteps, one-two, one-two—there is a rhythm to them. I feel my mother's face coming close to me. I am not looking at her face. She says: "Hold on to Maria. Take good care of her." There are tears in her voice. I have seen them on her face. I am only five and a half. I am falling apart. My legs, my arms, and my head are falling off. I hold myself very stiff. I push her face out of my eyes. I am still falling apart. But then—

I take my sister's hand,
I feel the pull of the pack on my back,
I touch my ribbon and feel its soft sound,
I see the little dancing lights on the soldiers' knives,
I know that I am not falling apart.

The soldiers march between the mothers and the children, and suddenly we are alone, with the soldiers behind us. I feel my mother's face. My sister is crying. My limbs are getting loose again. But—

I clutch my sister's hand,
I feel the pack on my back,
I touch the ribbon and hear the sound, I am together again.

We have to walk on. The train is hissing. It smells of smoke. The steps of the train are high and the knapsack pulls me back. I am holding on to my sister. We are in a compartment full of children. They cry. The door is slammed closed. The train jerks and moves. I do not know where we are going. My limbs are breaking again.

I clutch my sister's hand,
I feel the pack on my back,
I touch my ribbon and feel the soft sound,
And there is the rhythm of the train: TCHUKETEE
    tchuketee, TCHUKETEE tchuketee,
I am whole again.

Again, the train stops. The doors are opened. It is very dark. There are no soldiers this time, but ladies with strange white hats. They talk, but I do not understand them. We all leave the train. The steps are high. My beret falls off my head and rolls away. I try to get it, but we are told to move on. I hold myself very stiff and scream, until someone gives me my beret. We walk in a long line and enter a large room in a big house. There are only a few lights on. There are long tables with soup on them. I do not like the smell and cannot swallow the soup.

There is no pack on my back,
There is no rhythm of the train,
I clutch my sister's hand and look at the buttons on my shoes.
I want to count them, but I can't.

We climb endless stairs. Then we are in a large room with many beds. There is a lot of crying. My sister cries too. Tears try to leave my eyes, but I close them long and hard. When I open them again, the tears do not know how to come out anymore.

THE WHOLE TIME we were in Holland, I never knew where I was and why I was there. It was only much later that I found out that we were there for the food. At the time, I found the whole situation totally incomprehensible. I did not miss my family, because I had no emotional attachment to them. What I kept looking for were the concrete things I had known at home, like the shiny light reflected from the brass trim on the stove, or the multicolored light coming through a stained-glass window in the house. I was confused, because

I was cut off from anything by which I oriented myself, from the environment that made me the person I was. When I lost that, I lost everything, and to keep myself from just disintegrating, I had to stop thinking altogether. I became nothing more than a stiff little body.

Only once do I remember connecting with my new environment. We were taken for a walk down to the beach. We walked in a row, and I was suddenly struck by a design in the sand. It was a beautiful, rippling pattern, created by the wind. I bent down, wanting to move my hands back and forth over it, but there was a voice that told me to continue walking. I missed that design. I longed to go back to feel it, but I was never allowed to sit on the beach by myself, and I have no memory of ever looking at the rippled sand again.

I also have no memory of the return home. After six weeks we went back, but things were not the same anymore. It was as if the whole pattern I had known had shifted. And the fact that something familiar had been taken from me so abruptly and completely meant that the once stable and dependable had become unpredictable. Even though it was seemingly restored to me, I had lost it.

Shortly after our return, my parents decided to leave Belgium for the duration of the war. My father was Dutch. Messages had somehow gotten through from his relatives, convincing him that the family would be better off in Holland, which was not at war. As it turned out, we never went back to Belgium to live. My father had lost his business and we had no home there anymore. By the time he was able to reestablish himself, we were settled in Holland.

Before we could leave Belgium, German soldiers came to our house and marked the things we would be allowed to take with us. The rest had to be left behind. I remember seeing black crosses everywhere, but I have no recollection of leaving our home. The next thing I remember is being on the train. At the border, we had to stand in line for a long time.

Every single piece of clothing, every handkerchief, anything that was in our luggage was held up to the light by the German soldiers to see if it contained anything forbidden, like a message or something.

Someone had given me a little holy picture on parchment which I used to look at for hours. I was always attracted to anything colorful that light could shine through. One soldier got ahold of my little picture and since he couldn't read what was written on it, he tore it into little pieces, right before my eyes. I still see those pieces flying around. I don't know what dying is, but it must be something like what I felt at that moment. Everything was gone, as if life itself didn't exist anymore. This was the only thing, the only treasure I had. Without it I was lost, I was nothing.

I must have been confused by the whole experience, the disappearance of my familiar surroundings, the train journey into the unknown, the loss of my treasure. My father got separated from us, and my mother must have been in a highly anxious state. But I didn't register any of this. Again, I was nothing but a walking zombie, absolutely stiff, unfeeling, unseeing, not taking in what was spoken around me.

Until my parents could establish a new home for us, our family was divided up among our relatives. My sister and my brothers went to stay with some aunts and uncles in one part of the country, my parents lived in a small apartment with relatives in The Hague, and I was placed with another aunt and uncle, also in The Hague. They had no children and spoke no French. On the weekends they took me over to my parents' place, but all of this back and forth made things harder for me, rather than helping me adjust. I was torn apart inside and totally confused.

I remember smelling something cooking, for example. I think it may have been a roast. I knew the smell from a different environment, but I didn't recognize it, because it did not fit into the new one. I ate it only so as not to attract attention. Although I knew who my father and mother were, they were lost to me, in a sense. I had lost them, together with the familiar environment of which they had been a part and to which they belonged. They were familiar strangers.

My aunt and uncle were kind people, and they tried to show me their love. But to me, being hugged was very, very painful. I was put into one of the bedrooms in a huge bed that stood in a kind of an alcove. I had no concept of family, but I knew that besides me, there were six more who somehow belonged together. I had no idea where they were. I'm sure that I was told, but I didn't take any of it in. When I was put to bed, I moved to the very edge of it, all the way to the wooden frame. When my aunt came to check on me, she put me back in the middle of the bed, but I always rolled back, because somehow, somewhere, there needed to be space for something that had been part of my life. My aunt never succeeded in keeping me in the middle of the bed. Whatever anxieties I might have had about the separation from the rest of my family I eliminated, as if by magic, by sleeping at the edge of the bed. As long as there was room for them, somehow things that I had lost would return to normal.

I had already learned to protect myself against most any traumatic experience and go deaf, blind, and mute at will, but I still had a very hard time defending against the emotions of other people, because they were unpredictable and not under my control.

I remember, for example, how during the winter my uncle took me skating on one of the frozen canals. Although I had no idea what skating was, I was not afraid when he put skates on my boots and told me to hold on to his coat. He was a strong skater, and I hung on to him with all my might. Somehow I lost my grip and ended up sliding into one of the holes that were cut into the ice to give the ducks and other waterfowl some access to the water. Luckily, I was pulled out before I slid under the ice. I was soaking wet and very cold but not afraid. My uncle found me after a while and took me home. My aunt must have been very upset. The worst part of my misadventure was the loving look on her face, as she ministered to me. I had to close my eyes so I would not have to see it.

Although I was totally bewildered by what was happening to me, I never asked any questions. I stayed in a world to myself. Quite by accident, I discovered a way of making myself feel safe again. I found a hiding place.

The dining room table had a heavy cover over it that hung down all the way to the floor. I discovered that when I crept under there, I was absolutely isolated in a small, dark space. I could peek out into the world, but people couldn't see me. I hid there several times, and every time it was harder to come out again. One day I realized that if I stayed there too long, I might not ever be able to come out again. I somehow knew that I was in acute danger. If I went into hiding again, something irreversible might happen to me. I did not associate this with dying, but I must have felt that I might kill something if I stayed under that table. So I gave up my safe place. I deprived myself of that small pleasure.

But I was in hiding in other ways, looking out at the world from within my glass bubble, as if through a one-way mirror. I remember, for example, standing outside the house, waiting for my aunt. There was a group of children playing nearby, and I became very interested in them. They spoke Dutch, which I did not understand at the time, so I listened to the foreign sounds they made and watched the way they moved and how the expressions on their faces changed. They looked one way when they played with one another, but when they talked with a woman they called *Moeder*, which means "mother" in Dutch, they would have a completely different look on their faces.

From the time I was very small, I had developed the ability to observe, and I remember noting this phenomenon and being fascinated by it. These were perfectly normal children from the neighborhood in normal relationships. I did not play with them, but I watched them intently, and I knew that what I saw was important and that I would be able to use it at some time. I clearly remember saying to myself: "I must watch children so I can help them later on." And once I had decided what I must do, a sort of peace came over me. I was seven years old.

My father found a job as a house painter six or seven months later. He made very little money, but my mother was eager to have us all together again. I have no memories of joy or happiness about being reunited with my family. In the new environment, they were strangers to me. We moved into a small house, the first of many we lived in. Before we were finally settled, we moved thirteen times. This was very dangerous for me, because as soon as I had found something to hold on to in the new house, we moved again and I was lost to me.

I decided that I needed something I could keep, that would stay the same, no matter what. Most of the houses we moved into had at least one window with colored glass in it. I loved it when the sun shone through the window and made colored patterns on the floor. This was something I could keep from one move to the next. In one house, some of the wallpaper had a rough surface and beautiful colors. I loved to touch things. Feeling their texture seemed to ease whatever was going on in me. I pulled off a tiny piece of this special wallpaper and held on to it, until we were settled in our last house, after my father had been able to establish a business of his own again.

My mother was very homesick, and as soon as armistice was declared, it was decided that we would spend the whole summer with relatives in Belgium. They lived in the country somewhere, and there was food available there. Travel was still very difficult. Railroad tracks, bridges, and roads between Holland and Belgium had been destroyed, so we had to change trains frequently, with long waits in between.

By the time we came to the border, where we had to leave the train yet again, my mother was very tired. We had another interminable wait for the next connection and we had already been travelling for hours. My youngest brother, Charles, was only four years old; the other two boys were six and seven. My sister Maria was ten. My mother was a very strong woman, but she needed to rest. We were sitting on the platform, around a small, round table with a top of polished stone. It must have been marble. I clearly remember the design of the smooth, cold surface.

My mother looked at me and said: "Jeanne, pay attention to your brothers and sister, so I can rest a little." Her voice had a special quality in it that went right through me. I will never forget that sound. She put her head on the table and closed her eyes. Panic struck me. How was I going to manage? There were so many things to keep an eye on. I quickly counted them. There were thirteen pieces in all. Some of them stayed in place, but others kept moving around.

I was almost nine years old, but I didn't see much difference between the things that stayed put, which was the luggage, and those that milled about—my brothers and sister—although the former were easier to keep track of. I counted and counted, and whenever something moved from its original place, I tried to move it back. I cannot remember how long my mother slept, perhaps only fifteen minutes, but to me it seemed like an eternity.

To me, this last little vignette is the most striking example that to some children with autism spectrum disorder, people are basically just animated objects. Yet clearly Jeanne's mother saw her as the most responsible and trustworthy of the children, proof of the extent to which this highly intelligent child was able to hide and compensate for her disabilities. Additionally, it may illustrate the need for sameness, in this case to keep things in the same constellation.

Resistance to change is typical for almost all children living with autism. Their experience resembles a picture in a kaleidoscope. If it is shaken, the pieces arrange themselves in a different and unfamiliar pattern. In the same way, any change in a situation or environment means that the relationship of people to each other is changed, and they themselves may appear different within their relationship to other pieces.

Other children, too, may find change difficult or anxiety producing. Young children often cling to what psychologists call "transitional objects," something familiar from one environment to provide a link to the new one, like the piece of wallpaper Jeanne carried. For children with autism, such familiar, known objects become crucial to help them survive change, while the rocking and other repetitive movements Jeanne talks about seem to have a hypnotic and therefore calming effect, like the repetition of a mantra.

What is highly unusual in the way Jeanne dealt with situations that threatened to overwhelm her was that even as a young child she realized the danger inherent in completely losing touch with reality if she gave in to the pull of hiding in an inner world, be it that of the wonderful sensation of floating she associated with the smell of roses, described in an earlier chapter, or the safety of being in permanent hiding under the table, described in this one.

School years in Holland

4

Now that the family was together again, we were sent to school. Going to school was not a new experience for me. I had gone to kindergarten while we were still living in Belgium, in a school run by nuns. I can still picture them in their gray habits, with big wimples on their heads, but I don't remember their faces. I never looked up. I only saw these gray shapes moving back and forth among the rows of children.

Among the things in the schoolroom were two little statues, one of St. Joseph, one of Mary. Every day, these were put on the desks of two children, St. Joseph on the desk of a boy, Mary on that of a girl. I was fascinated with these statues and would have loved to touch them, but we were not allowed to walk around, and for some reason my desk was never selected.

I was also struck that whenever children got the statue, the expression on their faces changed. I watched them carefully and then I tried to form that same expression on my own face. I did this for hours, until my cheeks hurt, but I did not seem able to arrange my muscles into what I now know was a smile. Finally, the teacher noticed my grimacing. She must have thought that I was making faces at someone. There was a scolding voice, and I was put in a corner, with my face toward the wall. I didn't understand what I had done wrong, but I also didn't feel particularly bad about it. I must have associated the experience with the statues. In any case, I erased them from my mind and from that time on never consciously noticed them again.

When we entered school in Holland we didn't speak Dutch, but like most children exposed to a foreign language, we picked it up quickly, and eventually even started speaking it with one another, although at home we still only spoke French. I did well in school, but that was nothing more than what was expected of us. My parents were much more insistent on our getting good marks in "zeal" and "conduct" than interested in high grades.

By observing my environment closely, I figured out what I had to do, both at school and at home, to avoid drawing attention to myself. At no time did anybody ever suspect that there was something wrong with me. My father was a very wise but quiet man. Perhaps it was in his nature to make no emotional demands. Perhaps he sensed something special in me. In any case, he never seemed to ask for a relationship with me. I never had to close off from him. He was neither a threat nor a comfort. He was just there, part of the environment, like a familiar, comfortable piece of furniture.

My mother was a different story. She was very busy with looking after the family, but she was also observant and very caring. Little by little, I had managed to build a strong wall around myself so that fewer and fewer things could ambush me, but I could not completely escape my mother's notice. She always seemed to know what we were doing. I had to give her some answers when she showed an interest in my activities. But I had already discovered where my real freedom lay: others could see and hear what I did and said. But nobody knew what I was thinking. Once I realized that, I felt completely free.

By the time I was six years old, I had developed a number of compulsive behaviors as protection against situations I could not predict or control and against the threats of change and the loss of a familiar object or environment. I used sight, touch, and sound to distract and calm myself: staring at the light reflecting off the shiny copper trimmings of a wood stove or streaming through colored-glass transoms, tracing patterns with eyes and fingers, touching and rubbing materials to feel their texture or produce a soothing sound. And to these I now added counting.

My seventh birthday was approaching, and somehow there was something scary associated with that number, something changed. I had heard that one could sin, once one was seven, and if one died, one would not go straight to heaven. Although I had no idea what any of this meant, I had to protect myself against the threat of change. I started counting to seven over and over again. I started to do all activities in sevens. I walked to school counting from one to seven, I chewed my food counting the bites and taking the last one when I reached seven. I drank in seven swallows. I dressed, washed my hands and face, counting to seven.

The most difficult was to reach our pew in time, when going to church. I had to be in place on the count of seven. I talked only when I had absolutely no other choice. I didn't want to draw attention to myself, so I only used the counting when things were more or less under my control and no one would notice my doing it.

On my next birthday, the magic number became eight; the year after, nine. I continued this compulsive behavior until I was twelve. Then I stopped. I had almost become a total prisoner of my compulsions. It took all of my freedom away and I knew that if I didn't break out, there would be no end to it and my life would become more and more constricted. So just like that, overnight, I gave up counting.

But there were still times when I was in danger of being overwhelmed by anxiety. I do not know what triggered such moments, but I needed a strong defense against them. For about a year after I had given up counting, I became self-aggressive whenever the threat of anxiety became too powerful. I had a belt with a shiny buckle, and I used it to hit myself with. I do not remember feeling any pain, yet lashing my back somehow seemed to loosen the stranglehold of the anxiety. Again, reason came to my rescue. I realized that it would be very easy for me to hit myself too hard and hurt myself to the point where injuries would be discovered and provoke questions and concern. I stopped hitting myself, but even today, I can still feel the easing of tension within me when I think of the belt hitting my back.

Among the children, I was considered the quiet, sober one, the one who could be relied upon, who did exactly as was told and who made no demands. My older sister was fun-loving and giddy and covered my silence with her incessant chatter. We complemented each other quite well. I kept her out of trouble by taking on the responsibility of getting her up in time, keeping our room neat, and, later, when we started going out to parties, making sure that she kept whatever curfew we had. I never thought that it was unfair that I was given more responsibilities than Maria. I knew neither envy nor jealousy.

But even though I went along, I never felt that I was part of a group. It was almost as if only my body was there somewhere, on the edge of things. And if I could avoid it, I did not even physically participate in the activities of the other children. I was especially leery of games, because there often was an element of surprise to them.

I remember one particularly frightening occasion when we played a trick on a visiting aunt. A black stocking was stuffed to resemble a leg. Everybody sat in a circle. One person had surreptitiously bent one of her own legs back and substituted the stuffed stocking, which stuck out from under her dress in a very realistic way. My aunt was invited to go around the circle and pull at every leg. Of course, the artificial one started coming out. It looked very real, as if she were actually pulling a person's leg off. I had seen the stocking being stuffed, but I also saw the leg come off. The contradiction between these two realities was so confusing and frightening that I almost fainted.

After that incident I closed myself off even more tightly, so that I wouldn't register things anymore and be ambushed like that again. I still participated in games, because not to do so would have gotten me noticed, but I walked through them like a zombie. I responded to what was said to me, so I did hear and understand what was expected, but I remained untouched. It was as if it was all happening outside of myself.

Surprises that were supposed to be treats were harder to protect against. They combined the elements of change and the unknown with the possibility of disappointment and loss—if something you allowed yourself to feel happy about didn't materialize for some reason. If the treat was in the form of a present, it also carried within it the almost intolerable burden of the giver's expectations.

Wrapped presents were especially hard to deal with for me. First, there was the uncertainty of not knowing what to prepare for: pleasure or disappointment. And then, one had to make sure to react in the right way. I knew that not to show gratitude or joy at a present would disappoint and hurt the person who had chosen it. But I was incapable of deception. So, every time I received a present I had to worry. What would happen if I didn't like it? How could I act so as not to lie and yet not upset anyone? I would have much preferred to just get an empty wrapped box as a present. Then, I could have enjoyed the pretty wrapping paper and the ribbon, and would not have had to face the ordeal of unpredictability.

IT WAS EXTREMELY IMPORTANT to me that the emotional climate in our house remain temperate. Any kind of upheaval that resulted in an emotionally charged atmosphere was hard for me to tolerate, and I was so overly sensitive to any kind of emotion in others that I picked up on the slightest inflection in a voice, especially in my mother's voice, and I noticed the most fleeting changes of expression in her face. I could still paint her face today as it looked at one moment or another, when she was worried, troubled, or upset.

We were very poor during the war and for some time after it. We never starved. We were never really hungry. My mother was an excellent manager and made a little go a long way. But we could not afford the things we used to have. I remember my sister once asking her for a certain kind of biscuit we used to have in Belgium. I think it was something like "lady's fingers." The look on my mother's face was terrible to me, as was her sad tone when she said: "You'll have to be patient. We will have it again later."

After that, I made sure that nothing I said would make her sad like that, so I would never again have to see her expression of sadness that she did not have more to give to her children. I solved the problem by eating very slowly, and if there were seconds, I still had food on my plate and so I didn't have to have any.

I managed to stay almost unnoticed. I was accepted, I walked home with one or another of my classmates, I was invited to their birthday parties and may have even stayed overnight with one, but I did not develop a special friendship with any of them. And when I did get a little closer to someone, it took very little for me to lose that connection again. I remember once, for example, I was invited to a meal at someone's house. I still spoke mostly French at that time, so I called it *diner*. They thought that was funny and laughed a little about it. I was confused. I didn't know what I had done wrong, and I was very hurt. So that somehow changed the experience. Something was lost before it could develop further.

I avoided any situation that could bring people too close to me, so I never complained about anything. As it turned out, this severely endangered my life on several occasions. On the whole we were a healthy family, and I was no exception. But when I was thirteen I started having a stomachache that became more and more severe. I did not say anything about it, although it continued off and on for weeks.

The entire school always went for a long nature walk on the last Friday of each month. On the day of the walk, the pain was so excruciating that I fell behind the others and sat down behind a tree, because I could not continue to walk.

That evening my parents went to visit some neighbors and they had asked the neighbors' teenage daughter to stay with us during that time. I remember going to my bedroom, because I felt very sick. The pain was almost unbearable, and I couldn't talk about it. The others wanted to play a game and needed me. When I did not respond, they came to fetch me. I had such a high fever by that time that I didn't make any sense. My sister must have realized that I was really sick and called my parents.

I was taken to the hospital and operated on the same night. I did not know what was happening to me. The only thing I remember is that I was put on a stretcher. My father, who came with me, said, "Don't cry, because it will upset your mother." So I didn't cry. In fact, I was not afraid, only confused. Everything seemed oddly distorted, probably because I had such a high fever. My appendix had come close to rupturing. For a long time, there was nothing, only pain. I took it day by day. I didn't get upset, I didn't cry. I kept myself together. I knew that I had been operated on, though not why. I never asked any questions, and then I came home and that was over.

This chapter in Jeanne's life vividly illustrates several characteristics that distinguish children with neurotypical development from those with autism spectrum disorder (ASD), who often remain mute, or have severe impairments in language, not because they are deaf but because they have cut themselves off from social interactions and relationships.

While sounds can be learned by imitation, they do not attain meaning without being part of a dialogue. In the same way, the young Jeanne struggled to reproduce a smile by imitation, without either understanding the meaning of it or being able to make a connection between the facial expression and an emotional state of her own.

Compulsive behaviors are also very typical for many autistic individuals, possibly because they serve a soothing function. It is very rare, however, that an obsessive person is able to spontaneously give up compulsive behaviors, although quite frequently, as in Jeanne's case, different types of compulsions serially replace one another. Compulsive, self-injurious behaviors are also not uncommon in individuals with extremely high anxiety or depression. The best known are cutting or biting as well as head banging to the point where children have to wear helmets to prevent brain injury.

And, finally, staying silent about what must have been excruciating pain may have had just as much to do with Jeanne's fear of drawing attention to herself and evoking emotions in others (which she would then have had to deal with) as with an inability to identify pain as an indication that something was wrong—a phenomenon often seen in individuals with ASD, as discussed earlier.

Illness

5

After grade school I went on to high school. I remember the last high school year when I was sixteen as the most fun-filled of my entire life. I think I laughed enough during that year to last me for the rest of my life. There were only eight girls in my class, and we were all full of high spirits and mischief. For some reason, there was a lot of illness going around that year. Perhaps there was a flu epidemic. In any case, most of our regular teachers were out, and we had a succession of substitute teachers who were not very experienced in the first place and who were also handicapped by not knowing us.

I remember one teacher whom we disliked because he was very bossy. He was also very bald. He affected a derby hat, and one day we got ahold of it and proceeded to fill it with the shavings of our lead pencils. The unsuspecting teacher put on his hat, and the next time he lifted it in greeting, his head was revealed looking like a speckled egg. We thought this insult to his dignity absolutely hilarious.

Another teacher had the habit of perching on our desks while lecturing. He was a nice man, but we felt that he was being somewhat too familiar, and we sprinkled the edges of the desks with chalk dust. To his embarrassment, the teacher left our classroom with white pants.

All of our pranks were pretty harmless, though, and the director couldn't really do too much to us, because we continued to work hard and get good grades. He eventually realized that what we needed was someone who could control us. He engaged an experienced man from Friesland who right from the beginning made it clear that he was going to stand no nonsense from us. So after about three months of fun and games, things returned to normal.

None of the subjects we were taught posed any real difficulties for me except composition. I had no problems as long as we were asked to write about real things or experiences. But I remember an exercise in which we were given one paragraph of a story and were expected to develop it into a full-length tale of at least two pages. Because of my lack of imagination, it was impossible for me to make up facts beyond those given in the text. I was incapable of making up anything the characters in such a tale might be doing or saying. I tortured my brain to at least come up with some additional adjectives to flesh out the descriptions given in the text. If a character was said to wear a sweater, for example, I labored to describe it in great detail, perhaps based on a sweater owned by someone I knew: the texture, the color, the stitching, or how warm it was. In this way, I was usually able to pull and push the paragraph into the minimum length required, and although I got barely passing grades, I managed to pass the course.

After graduating from secondary school at sixteen, I entered the equivalent of teachers training college, where I was enrolled in a two-year course, leading to a degree in early childhood education.

When I was seventeen and about a year away from receiving my diploma, an epidemic of diphtheria broke out. One of my brothers got it and was hospitalized. The health department advised all parents to have their children inoculated. My mother was initially against it, but she gave in when the doctor told her that if my baby sister should catch the illness she would not survive. The Red Cross had opened an inoculation center, and there were long lines of people waiting to get their shots. In all, three shots were necessary, and at that time they were given between the shoulder blades.

Something went wrong with my last injection. The needle hit a spot in my spine and broke off. It hurt so much that I could feel the pain from my head all the way down my back. The needle was pulled out, but after a while I started to feel sick. I developed headaches, and soon they became almost unbearable. I also had stiffness and pain in my neck and down my back.

As usual, I told nobody. Every day, I went off to school on my bicycle. It was a thirty-minute ride and I knew that there was something wrong, because I started to have slight accidents on my bicycle. I couldn't seem to stay on a straight line. I hit trees and veered off the path. I had developed double vision, so I saw two trees where there was one. It was also harder and harder to stay awake. Studying became impossible. I fell behind in every subject. One day I fell asleep in class. The teachers noticed that I was unwell, and I was told to stay home until I felt better. I was caught in a dilemma. I could no longer go to school, but I also couldn't stay home, because then I would have to tell my mother about my problems and she would worry.

Every morning, at the regular time, I left home, but instead of going to school, I went to the woods. I stayed there until school let out and then went home. At home, I spent all my time in my room. My mother thought I was studying. Mealtimes were difficult. I had no appetite, and my double vision made it hard to serve myself and to handle my utensils properly. I heard family friends remark that I looked awful, but my mother explained that I was studying hard for my final exams.

My symptoms got worse. My balance became poor, and my left arm and leg felt weak. My main worry, however, was to find ways to hide my condition from my family. September 28 was my mother's birthday. That afternoon, several friends and family members had come over to celebrate with her. There may have been only eight people in all, but when I got home there seemed to be unbelievably large crowd in the room. The pain in my head, neck, and back was excruciating. I tried to escape upstairs, but I was dizzy and off balance, and I couldn't make it. I leaned against the living room door and broke down. I had to tell my mother about my pain.

She called the doctor, who had me come to his office. He lived on the other side of the town, and I had to take a streetcar. I went alone. I still do not know how I made it. When I came to the terminal, I had to cross several tram lines and a street to get to the doctor's office. It took me forever to cross. Every streetcar was multiplied. I saw nothing but weaving tram rails.

The doctor realized immediately that there was something seriously wrong with me. He sent me home by taxi and told my mother to keep me in bed until a neurologist could examine me. When the specialist made his house visit the next day, he was surprised to hear my mother tell him that I had been fine up to the day before. He was puzzled by my condition and ordered complete bed rest. I was glad to be in bed, but I had to find a way to avoid worried faces and voices. I asked for books and also offered to watch my baby sister while my mother did the housework. Of course, I could not read, and having the baby with me was pure torture. Also, I did not get better by staying in bed. Every move made my head hurt worse.

When the doctor returned after a few days, my mother told him that I must be feeling better, since I had been reading and playing with my baby sister. He examined me again and then suggested that I come to the clinic for observation. My mother, not knowing how ill I was, took me there by streetcar and bus. It was a journey of one hour. I don't know how I survived it.

Once I was in the hospital and in bed, I stopped fighting. I no longer had to hide that I was in pain to avoid my family's worried faces. I was being taken care of by strangers. I remember little of the first few months in the hospital. I had several painful neurological examinations. My left arm and leg had become practically useless and my eyesight was deteriorating. I could hardly see and I slept most of the time. For a while I thought that I was in a dark room. I must have been blind for a while. I was told later that I also had long periods of unconsciousness.

One day I heard two doctors talking together. I was not aware of my body, but I remember one of them saying "If she lives at all, she will take at least eighteen months to recuperate, but she will always be paralyzed and blind."

"That's what you think," I thought, and blacked out again.

During one of my lucid moments, I asked the doctor what had happened to my left arm and leg. He patted my shoulder and told me not to worry, but he didn't give me any explanations. Sometime later I woke up and found myself lying in a deep, padded, boxlike bed in a small room. I was totally disoriented. When the doctor came, I begged him to take me back to my familiar room. I asked him why I was in that box, but again, he only patted my shoulder and gave some meaningless exhortation not to worry. I asked a nurse and the priest who visited the hospital to tell me what was going on. I wanted to know what was happening to me, why I couldn't move the limbs on my left side, but no one gave me any explanation. It was only years later that I learned that I had had encephalitis and that I had had severe seizures during the worst part of my illness.

Very slowly, I seemed to be getting a little better. I still had seizures and would suddenly fall asleep at odd times, but I was alert most of the time. Some of my sight had come back, although my arm and leg did not improve. I had to stay flat on my back. Only at mealtimes the nurse would raise my head.

After a while, I discovered that I could move some of the fingers of my left hand very slightly. I also thought that I had a little feeling in my left leg. I told the doctor, who did several tests and then said that I was mistaken. I was resigned to being nearly blind. I had very acute hearing and thought that it could make up for the loss of sight. I could identify people the way they walked and could tell time almost to the minute. But not being able to control my body bothered me. It meant that I would have to depend on others, possibly for the rest of my life. Something had to be done.

With my hands under the blanket, I exercised my fingers and also massaged my left leg. By the time spring came around the seizures were almost under control. The weather was beautiful, and I asked if I could not be put outdoors. The doctor gave his permission and I was rolled out into the woods on a stretcher. First a nurse stayed with me, but eventually I was left alone for a while. This was my chance to do something for my leg. I was sure that if there was some life left in it, it would not be good for it to keep it immobilized for such a long time.

One day, after the nurse had left, I managed to roll over on my stomach and to swing my legs over the edge. Hanging on to the stretcher with my right arm and putting my weight on my right leg, I touched the ground with the toes of my left foot. I thought that I could feel it. With great difficulty, I maneuvered myself back onto the stretcher. I was exhausted but satisfied. I repeated this exercise whenever I was left alone, trying to put a little more weight on my toes every time. In bed, after the lights were out, I moved my left leg with my right hand, up and down, up and down. My leg felt as if it were made out of lead, but almost imperceptibly it got stronger. One day after I had climbed off the stretcher, I lifted the right foot and for a split second my left leg supported me. I did not tell anyone about this, not because I meant to be secretive, but because it simply did not occur to me that they needed to know.

In the meantime, the doctor had asked my parents for permission to try an experimental drug on me. I was told only that I would be given injections for six weeks and that I would have to stay in bed, because the medicine would cause me to have a fever. The liquid in the injections looked like iodine. The injections were very painful, and if the doctor missed the vein in my arm, it felt as if fire was going into it. I felt sick most of the time, and my arms were bruised. As predicted, I got a fever, which rose steadily for three weeks and then slowly subsided. After six weeks of this treatment, the doctor felt that there was some improvement. My arm and leg were somewhat stronger. Personally I thought this improvement was due to my exercises, but I did not enlighten him.

I was allowed to go outside again and I continued exercising my leg and made real progress. But after another six-week period, the injections were to be resumed. The new bottle from which the liquid was drawn was about the size of a jelly jar. The first injection made my heart race, and I felt as if I was going to faint. The director of the clinic was told of my reaction to the treatment and gave me the second injection himself. My heart started to race again and then it seemed to stop. Just before I passed out I heard the doctor curse and yell for oxygen. It turned out that they had made the mistake of not diluting the mixture properly. When I came to, I was in an oxygen tent and was told to lie very still and not to move. It was three weeks before I was able to sit up again.

After a while I tried to get out of bed when the nurse was out of the room. By hanging onto the bed, I was able to move around it, and although I had most of my weight on the right leg, my left leg seemed able to support me just a little. When the nurse caught me in this activity, I insisted that I could walk, if she supported me. She ordered me back into bed, but told the director about my activities. I pleaded with him to let me practice, and at last he gave his permission. He suggested that we put a brace on my leg, but I refused.

At first it took two nurses to support me, but after a while I managed with one. I made real progress, and the doctor was convinced that it was all due to his treatment. My arm, too, had regained quite a bit of strength, so I asked for two canes. I wanted to try to walk by myself. I had to be very persistent, but eventually they let me try it. After that, I made rapid progress.

I had been in the hospital for about a year when suddenly I got a strong urge to go home for a visit. It was not a desire to see my family; it was an almost irresistible force without any particular feeling to it. I told the nurse that I *had* to go home. She replied that it was not to be thought of. I insisted. She called the doctor. He told me that I was not well enough to travel anywhere, that it would be too strenuous and dangerous for me. I could not give him a convincing reason, but I also knew that nothing could prevent me from going. At last he granted me a few hours leave and ordered a taxi for me.

At home, they were extremely surprised to see me. I asked after everyone and was told that they were all well except Maria, who had an infected arm. She had apparently cut herself while opening a can of sardines. I asked to see her arm and discovered that it was in terrible shape. It was red and infected and swollen from the hand to over the elbow. She was also running a fever. She had apparently been taken to the doctor the day before, but since then, her arm had become worse.

I stayed home for no more than fifteen minutes. I told my mother that I would take my sister to the hospital with me to have her arm looked at. My mother looked puzzled, but she let us go. She was a strong-willed woman and not usually that passive. But she must have been struck by my determination. At the hospital, I handed my sister over to the doctor. I was told to get back into bed and did so. I felt quite calm again and did not give the whole incident another thought. Sometime later a surgeon came to my room and told me that I had probably saved my sister's arm. One more day without treatment and it would have been too late.

I cannot remember that anyone in my family ever mentioned my strange behavior until a few years ago, when my sister asked me if I remembered how I had saved her arm. She wondered how I knew that she had been hurt. I gave her some vague answer. The truth is that this was not the first time something like that had happened to me, nor was it to be the last.

I dislike talking about this phenomenon, because I cannot explain it intellectually and I have no control over it. I do not like being taken over in this way and tried to fight it as I grew older, but it has come in useful on several occasions, when I was able to prevent serious accidents or, as in the case of my sister, when it saved her arm.

During the last eight months in the hospital, I asked for my books. My eyes had gotten strong enough so that I could read, and I wanted to make up for lost time. The doctor told my mother that I would never be able to study again. He thought that there had been too much damage done by my illness, but again he gave permission, when I insisted. He was sure that I would discover my limitations soon enough by myself.

What I did discover was that I could not remember names. Sometimes I did not even remember the names of family members or friends. I solved that problem by connecting names with objects I knew or could see. I never totally regained a memory for names. Especially when I am under great stress, I lose them. When I was suddenly separated from my family and my country, during World War II, for example, I forgot even the names of my sisters and brothers and the name of my hometown. Looking at an atlas, I said the name out loud, to fix it again in my memory. But seeing a name in writing was not enough. I had to hear the sounds associated with it as well.

Luckily, I had not lost the ability to conceptualize. But the most important thing I had going for me was infinite patience and the capacity to concentrate. It was a long struggle, but I did not get frustrated. I never had any doubts that I would eventually achieve what I was looking for. I accepted the fact that I had sustained some brain damage, but I also knew that only a small part of the brain's capacity is ever used, and I was determined to develop my brain's capacity to make up for the losses I had sustained.

During the last few months of my hospital stay I was moved to the convalescent center, where I had a lot more freedom. I still had to rest a certain number of hours every day and could not leave the grounds without permission. There was some concern about occasional seizures, but I took full advantage of my freedom. I found an old bicycle in a shed on the grounds and used it to exercise with. At first I just sat on it, letting my feet touch the ground and slowly propelling myself forward that way. After a lot of practice I could ride for a few seconds, and by the time the doctors had decided that they could do no more for me, I was able to wobble along a little. But it took a good year before I regained sufficient balance to ride safely again.

I had been away from home for two years, and when I returned, everything was unfamiliar. My older brothers had visited me a few times in the hospital, yet they seemed to be complete strangers. They were adolescents now. They had learned to dance; they played tennis, went sailing, and had parties. My older sister had become engaged. I think my family felt uncomfortable with me. They had been told about my seizures and that I would not be able to continue with an education. But I did not let anyone else's opinions deter me. I simply announced that I would go back to school. My mother did not encourage me, but she also put up no objections. I do not think that she could have stopped me.

As I was beginning to feel stronger, I began to go out more and become involved again with activities organized by my family. For a while I was also active in a Catholic youth group that had been founded to counteract the growing influence of communist youth cells that were beginning to attract a lot of youngsters. My sister was a very sociable young woman, and both of us were frequently invited to parties at the homes of family friends. We went on picnics and other outings and participated in all the other activities our circle organized, although I could no longer participate in sports, except for sailing, which I enjoyed a great deal.

There was one young man, the son of a well-to-do business family, who started to single me out and frequently invited me to go on rides with him. In those days, it was rare for young people to have a car of their own. I loved to ride in his car, and we went sailing together, went out to dinner, and attended parties. He was fun to be with, he had a big heart and I found him attractive. We seemed to agree on many things. He, too, loved children, and we had some vague plans of perhaps one day opening a school together. Before I knew it, we seemed to be engaged.

I never really thought about what that meant. We had an engagement party and received all sorts of presents. What I remember most vividly was my pleasure in seeing the sunshine through a set of crystal glasses we were given. The rainbow colors of the deflected light reminded me of the way the sun had shone through the colored glass and had dappled the floor around me when I was a small child. I did not think beyond the present, and if marriage was mentioned, I imagined at most the ceremony in church I was familiar with.

It took me a year of hard work to graduate with a degree in early childhood education. Then I spent two further years getting trained in the Montessori method, which was quite new then and interested me. I was twenty-two years old when I got my first job.

Jeanne often stressed that she never gave much thought to the physical part of intimacy. It didn't worry or concern her. She liked this young man who shared her interests and with whom she could imagine someday starting a school of their own. However, she was not in love with him. Indeed, she said that she had no clue what people meant when they talked about being in love. There was no emotional connection beyond shared interests and shared good times. The concept of "marriage" for her was defined by concrete events, such as getting presents and the outward ritual of the marriage ceremony.

As it turned out there was no marriage, partly because World War II intervened. Jeanne did not seem to have had any regrets about this. In fact, as she repeatedly told me when we talked about marriage or love relationships, and as she writes in chapter 13, she could not have survived in the kind of emotional intimacy that marriage demands or expects.

After our book *The Hidden Child* had been published, Jeanne regretted that we had not included a chapter on how to deal with children with autism when they fell ill. From her own experiences and especially her strong aversion to evoking emotions in others and being fussed over, she had developed the theory that a factual approach, with straightforward explanations of what needed to be done, was best. This is, of course, difficult for caregivers to understand and follow, especially parents, most of whom are naturally concerned, caring, and intent on comforting a sick child.

The teacher

6

For the next seven years, Jeanne used her teacher training in a variety of settings. I have condensed those experiences in this chapter. They are of interest because her early work already contains all of the elements of the novel teaching methods she later applied to international acclaim at Linwood.

Peter

I always knew that I wanted to work with children, especially at the preschool level. But I never particularly wanted to teach in a classroom. Just as I finished my education, there was a family that had heard I was looking for a job. Their only son, Peter, who was about six years old at the time, refused to go to school, so they were looking for a tutor for him. The challenge intrigued me, and I accepted.

I quickly discovered that Peter was determined not to learn. He refused to do anything that looked like work. He did not answer the simplest questions and lacked the most basic knowledge. He did not know his colors or numbers, for example, yet I had the impression that he was an intelligent child. I realized that I would have to approach teaching him in a roundabout way, so at first we just played. This also gave me an opportunity to discover what he was interested in, and almost against his will he started learning a few things through play.

The breakthrough came when I was able to make use of his love for babies. He knew that I had a baby sister, and he asked whether she could come to visit. He was eager to share his toys with her and to introduce her to his sandbox, which was his favorite place to play out of doors. But every time he played in it, he ended up urinating in it. It was not as if he wasn't completely toilet trained. It was just that the little puddle he created seemed to give him great satisfaction.

I had not previously tried to stop him. First of all, I didn't want to get into a power struggle with him; but I also figured it was his sandbox and his urine. I didn't have to play in it, and if needs be, the dirty sand could easily be cleaned out and replaced. I just bided my time, knowing that sooner or later I could use this in some way.

When he wanted my little sister to join him in the sandbox, I said, "Peter, you know there is that spot where you urinate, what about that?" He tried to dismiss my concern by saying that the wet spot would dry. I admitted that this was true but reminded him that it smelled and told him that I didn't want my baby sister to be sitting in that place accidentally. We thought about that for a while, and then I suggested that perhaps we could build a little fence around the spot, so we would know where it was. He agreed that this was a good idea.

I happened to have a large box of colored crayons and proposed to use these as the fence posts. I discussed with him how to mark the limits of the spot. I counted out four crayons of the same color and had him use these as the corner posts. Then we started filling in the sides, using a different color for each side and counting how many crayons were needed to fence in the whole area. With his interest engaged, he forgot his resistance to learning and quickly picked up knowledge of colors and numbers.

Since my sister came several times, we had to rebuild the fence, and Peter remembered how many crayons it took to make it and what colors to use. When I suggested a shortcut, it made sense to him that instead of counting each crayon, we could add groups of them, according to color. So we counted, and added, and from there progressed to multiplying, all within a relatively short time. I expressed concern that we might forget the exact number of crayons needed and that it might be useful to write them down. So he learned to write numbers and letters: so many yellows, so many reds, and before he knew it, he was doing arithmetic. In order to decipher what I dictated to him, he also had to learn to read, single words at first, longer sentences by and by.

At first all these activities centered on those crayons and the visits from the baby, but after a while, we included other things he was interested in. There had obviously been nothing wrong with him other than that he was overprotected, spoiled, and immature. As the only child of wealthy parents, he had had a nanny and a governess, but nobody had ever asked anything of him or challenged him in any way. By accepting him as he was, and by using what he was interested in, I was able to disarm his resistance to learning. I didn't ask him to do anything, or give up anything he wasn't ready for, not even urinating in the sandbox. I simply helped him to limit this behavior by literally fencing it in.

After a year I felt that Peter was ready for entry into a regular school. I also thought that he needed to be with other children. His parents saw the strength of my arguments and agreed to send Peter to school. He did very well there, and I heard that he eventually became a successful man.

Christine

My next pupil was Christine, the seven-year-old daughter of well-to-do parents, whose odd looks and behavior had kept her out of public school. Because of her retarded development, she had been isolated from outside contacts and had never had any formal schooling. In many ways her features resembled those of children with Down syndrome, but as I got to know her better, it seemed to me that her lack of knowledge was in good part due to her adamant refusal to be taught, rather than to an innate lack of intelligence. She was willful and had been overindulged, but I sensed that there was more to her than met the eye.

She was no more willing to be taught by me than she had been by anyone else, but we got along, which is more than can be said about her relationship with most other people. At first we simply spent a lot of time together out of doors, going for long walks, which we both enjoyed. On one of those walks, she suddenly snapped at me: "Don't push William against the wall." I apologized, saying that I hadn't seen William and asked who he was. It turned out that William was an invisible companion. In fact, Christine informed me, he was her husband. I apologized again for my clumsiness but reminded her that she had never introduced me to William.

When I showed my interest, Christine told me more about William, and at one point I asked her whether he was intelligent. Christine proudly asserted that William knew everything.

From then on, I started to include William in my attempts to teach Christine. I never pretended that I could see him or that he existed for me, but I accepted that he was real for her. Instead of asking Christine for an answer, I often asked William's help instead. I would tell him, for example, that I wasn't quite sure of the answer to a math problem I had introduced Christine to. And almost invariably, William knew the answer.

William became my entry into Christine's mind. By including and challenging him, I got her to participate in our lessons. She could not admit that William did not know something. He was perfect. On the occasions when she couldn't answer for him, she let me know that William didn't feel like talking just then. That told me that I had gone too fast with something and was asking too much of her. I could then go back over the material and ease her into it more slowly. In this way, she learned without protest and made rapid progress. I quickly realized that far from being retarded, she was in fact unusually intelligent. However, she continued to resist when asked to sit at a desk to write anything, and she refused to do any kind of homework. For quite a while, all of our work together had to be done outside.

A room had been set aside for our exclusive use, and whenever we came in from one of our walks, Christine would play school. She was the teacher, and she had a class of about twenty-four imaginary pupils, all of whom had names and had their assigned places. She seemed to remember each of them and called on them in turn. I was so intrigued that I secretly wrote down the seating arrangement and discovered that she never made a mistake. She never confused their names and she never forgot which pupil sat where. To these children, Christine taught what she had learned each day. To do that, she naturally had to write on the board, and in this way, she repeated everything I had written down for her. William was there and helped her, and her progress accelerated to the point where she could be integrated into a group home.

St. Vincentius

I was approached by one of the board members of St. Vincentius, a Catholic institution near Leyden, a small town near Amsterdam. It was for children whose parents had been considered unfit to look after them. Some of the parents were prostitutes or pimps, others alcoholics, and some were in jail for various crimes.

St. Vincentius housed between sixty and seventy youngsters, some only infants. At fourteen, the boys would be apprenticed to some tradesman and would leave the institution, while girls went into service at age eighteen. They were housed in separate wings of the building and were kept strictly apart. They were allowed no contact with each other, even though some of the children had brothers or sisters in the same institution.

I was originally hired to supervise the older girls, but shortly after I arrived the person in charge of the youngest children left, and they were given into my care also. So here I was, twenty-three years old, in sole charge of thirty-three children between the ages of three months and eighteen years of age and on duty twenty-four hours a day! Because St. Vincentius was a charitable institution, there was very little money, and I was only paid a token stipend, perhaps the equivalent of ten dollars a month.

St. Vincentius was housed in a large stone building next to the parish church and close to the school the children attended. Apart from the dining room, which doubled as a living room, there was only a large dormitory under the eaves and a kitchen. Except for the absolute necessities of a table and chairs in the dining room and cots in the dormitory, there was little furniture, and what there was was miserably inadequate.

The wooden chairs in the dining room had contraptions nailed against the backs so as to force the children to sit up straight. It made leaning back not only uncomfortable but painful. I took one look at these instruments of torture, found a hatchet, and hacked them off singlehandedly. This caused some consternation, but the protest didn't bother me, and the chairs stayed unadorned.

The iron cots in the attic had thin mattresses. A few had a whole blanket, but on most, the covers consisted only of the remnants of four or five pieces, worn thin by use. In the middle of the attic there was a small cubicle partitioned off by flimsy walls that did not extend to the ceiling. It had just enough space for a single bed, a washstand, a chair, and a rod to hang up some clothes. This was to be my room. A three-month-old baby had to temporarily sleep in my cell with me, which meant that the only way for me to get dressed was to sit on the bed.

The children went to school both morning and afternoon, coming back for the main meal of the day at noon. It usually consisted of mashed potatoes into which was mixed some other vegetable, such as carrots, cabbage, or spinach. This mush was mostly flavored by lard. Occasionally, slivers of meat were added to it. A glass of milk completed the meal. The children usually got another mug of tea after school, and supper was two slices of black bread, one with lard, one with a slice of some cold cut, accompanied by more tea.

St. Vincentius was a church foundation, governed by a board of directors, all Catholic citizens of Leyden, who set policy and hired the staff. In the past they had always hired people whose only qualification was that they were devout Catholics. This led to a frequent turnover of staff, unable to cope with these children, many of whom had been abandoned, neglected, or abused by their parents.

I soon discovered that the spirit that governed St. Vincentius was anything but charitable. The governors truly believed that the sins of the fathers are visited on the children. Because of who their parents were, these children were considered to have bad blood, and the only way to save them was to chastise them. The board went to great lengths to do this. Corporal punishment was commonplace. Upon my arrival I had been given a switch, which was to be used at the slightest sign of disobedience, such as being late for anything or talking back to staff. I was told that I was going to be held responsible for the children's behavior as well as their work. I was to get them up for church and make sure they got to school on time. The first thing I did was to throw away the switch. It could not help them or me. The director disapproved. She was sure the board would not like it. The only way to get through to them and to keep them under control, she said, was to hit them. I told her that if I could not gain the children's confidence and trust with love and understanding, I would not stay, so for the time being we were at a standoff.

It was also believed that working was good for the soul, and almost all the work, except for the cooking, was done by the children. After school, even the little girls were sat down with a pile of the black woolen stockings they all wore to be mended.

The older girls helped with the laundry, boiled in large copper kettles in the washhouse, hung out on lines, and ironed with heavy irons made of solid metal. They also had to scrub the floors, help in the kitchen, and do the more difficult mending. They left school at age fourteen and were trained to go into domestic service at age eighteen. The children had no toys and were given no time to play. Even after supper, they were kept busy with chores until their bedtime at nine.

Before I was hired, staff and directors had come and gone in quick succession, mainly because the girls had made life impossible for them.

When I introduced myself to them, they looked at me with cold dislike and contempt. I heard them whisper to each other "We'll get rid of her, too." I looked at these children dressed in drab, outdated clothes that didn't fit, in heavy black stockings and worn-down shoes, and my heart went out to them. They were innocent victims, stigmatized by society because of the mistakes their parents had made. They had never been taken care of by anyone, they were unloved and abandoned, and they repaid society with hostility and suspicion for its treatment of them. Somebody had to care. Somebody had to see the human beings in them. I had to find a way to understand and reach them.

I was in trouble the very first morning. When it was time to get up, the older girls did not stir. I proceeded to dress the smaller children and then went from bed to bed, touching the girls gently and reminding them that it was really time to get up. They seemed surprised and somewhat confused by this approach and got out of bed. "Tomorrow she will yell at us like all the others," I heard them say to each other. The next day, it took a little longer to get them up. They waited for me to get impatient, but I had unlimited patience, and they did not succeed in provoking me into a show of anger. Several days later they asked me why I didn't use the switch. I told them that I had thrown it away, because I didn't believe in hitting children and didn't know how to use a switch. That puzzled them.

One day, they decided to go "on strike." The older girls had to take turns scrubbing the dormitory floor. When I did my rounds, I found the girl who was supposed to do the work that week stretched out on her stomach, reading a book on sex she had smuggled in. Instead of upbraiding her, I asked to see the book and then told her that I had something much better on the subject and offered to lend it to her. If she was surprised at my reaction, she covered it with a sneer: "It's probably a holy book." But when I went to fetch it, she accepted it and had to admit that it was not too bad. "It even has pictures in it," and she plunked herself down and proceeded to read it.

I put on the wooden shoes that were worn for doing housework and proceeded to scrub the floor. After a while of trying to ignore this, the girl began to fidget. She looked at me, clearly discomfited, and asked whether I was going to finish the whole floor. I told her that I really didn't have a choice. It had to be done. However, if I was doing her work for her, I would not have time to do my own. This meant that she had to do my job. "Oh no," she said, "I don't want your job," and she went back to her scrubbing. In the afternoon, the girls who helped in the kitchen went on strike. I told the cook not to worry. I would do their job and they could do mine. That was the end of that strike!

There was a big uproar a few days after "the strike." The girls had broken into some locked cabinets and had "stolen" food. They had also taken cookies and candy from the executive director's room. She showed me the closet they had broken into, and I was surprised to see several large tins full of cookies. I asked why she had so many sweets, and she told me that they were for the children—whenever they deserved them. Apparently no one had deserved any for a long time. I really could not blame the girls for trying to get some extra food, although I couldn't sanction their breaking into cabinets to get it. How was I to deal with this situation? I hoped and prayed to have a solution before the end of the day.

In the evening, I found a few minutes to go to the village and bought all the plums I could afford to with what money I had. I put them in a bowl in the middle of the table in our little corner, and waited for the girls to come down. It took a long time. They obviously expected to be punished. At last they entered the room very reluctantly and sat down, not saying a word. It was a nice evening, and the window was open. Just at the right time, the maintenance man, who lived on the property with his wife, came by. He was a very nice man. He leaned in through the open window to exchange greetings, and when he saw the plums, he said: "The girls must have been extra good today to deserve such a treat." I sighed and said "Yes, I guess they were." The girls all started talking at once: "No we were not. Why do we get this?" I told them that I had not been able to think of anything else to do, but that before they started eating the plums, I would like them to talk about why they had done what they did, what was on their minds.

I learned a lot about them that evening. They talked about their homes. They thought of their home and their parents in very unrealistic, glorified ways. Some had been in institutions since they were toddlers. I asked them whether they knew why they had been removed from their homes. Most did not. I tried to explain to them that their parents had made mistakes, that they had not known how to take care of them, perhaps because many of them had themselves grown up in institutions. I answered all their questions about their parents as honestly as I could. I also promised them that I would try to visit their homes to give them more accurate information about their parents. I also told them that it was up to them to break the cycle, that they had the power to better themselves and to make sure that their own children would not end up in institutions. They promised not to "steal" anymore. In turn, I promised that I would continue to do anything I could to make their lives more comfortable, but told them that I would need their cooperation. Then they ate the plums.

I know that after that night they trusted me. I had been honest with them. But how to keep my promise to them? The first thing I had to do was to see to it that they got a better diet.

Several of the girls suffered from boils, and I was sure their diet was to blame. The staff and the executive director ate in a separate little room. Here, the meals were very good. One day, I asked why the children did not get more fruit, meat, and butter or margarine instead of lard. I got the same answer I was always given when trying to make some improvements: that the children did not deserve to be "coddled," that what they were getting was good enough for them. I insisted, and at last the director promised to make some changes.

I waited patiently, but nothing happened. I decided to take matters into my own hands. On the day of the next board meeting, I set aside some of the food that had been served to the children at noon. The board met in a special room with a cloth-covered table and comfortable chairs. No one was ever allowed in there except for the executive director and board members. When the meeting was in session, I marched into the room and put a plate with the food on it in front of each board member. They were stunned at my appearance in their sanctum and could not believe what was happening.

It was the first time I had seen the board together like this. They were mostly elderly men, sober city fathers, very much aware of their influence and importance, all sitting stiffly around the table. I did not apologize for my breach of the conventions but asked them to taste the food. As if mesmerized, they did. They said nothing, simply continued to stare at me. I told them that the children's health was at stake if they did not receive more adequate food, and I outlined what I wanted for them. They listened and then promised more fat and meat and fruits in season. Then I picked up the plates and left the room. Throughout, the executive director had looked as if she would have liked to vanish under the table. There had been much shaking of heads among the governors, but there was no talk of firing me. The first battle was won.

The next step was to get warm capes for the schoolchildren and for the little ones. Once upon a time the capes they wore had been black, of warm, thick wool. But over the years they had become so worn out that they were green and threadbare. They provided no warmth whatsoever. Once again, I invaded a board meeting. I held the capes up to the light. You could practically read through them. I guess that by now the governors had gotten used to my tactics. Although I never got a smile of approval, their sternness had dissipated somewhat. I got the new, warm capes for the youngsters.

Although I had not been aware of it, the board had begun to look into the situation at St. Vincentius a little more closely. They could not understand the lack of decent food. The executive director had not misappropriated any money, but she was obviously a poor manager, and the enterprise was in the red. It was finally decided that the institution should be taken over by a religious order that had convents nearby, nuns to run the girls' side, brothers to supervise the boys. The existing staff was dismissed. Only I was asked to stay on. It seemed that the nuns liked me, and the girls had been very upset at the idea of my leaving, so I promised to continue working there for a while longer.

The nuns were wonderful. They were kind and patient and quickly gained the confidence of the girls. I told them about all the changes I had made and outlined the future improvements I had in mind. After two intense years, I could close this chapter of my life with a good feeling.

Jeanne did follow up on her promise to visit the girls' homes to give them more accurate information about their parents and among other improvements even managed to get permission to have parents come and visit with their children.

Jeanne's next job found her in radically altered circumstances. She was engaged by an aristocratic family as a governess for their two older daughters, who at the time were three and five.

The little countesses

The count was German but had become a Dutch citizen. The countess was French. At home the family only spoke French, but it was important to them that the children become proficient in a number of languages early on.

I was expected to live in, since in France a governess almost takes the place of the mother.

The parents were abroad a lot and saw the children mostly when they were in Holland, and even then by appointment only. Most days, the girls were summoned to their parents' bedroom while the parents were having their breakfast. After about fifteen minutes, they were dismissed again. Sometimes the countess, who loved gardening, would invite the children to help her in the garden.

I had complete freedom in how to educate the children. I did not want to push them, but they were so intelligent, they learned very quickly. Most of the day we spoke Dutch, but during recess they were allowed to speak French. In the beginning I kept instructional periods short, but teaching also went on outside our formal lessons, through play, songs, and stories. It continued even when we were traveling. Everything we saw and did somehow lent itself to teaching.

Around the following Easter, I was asked whether I would mind accompanying the children to Paris, where they were to stay with their grandmother for an extended visit.

The grandmother was very beautiful, with skin that reminded me of alabaster. Every day I had to report to her on the work I was doing with her granddaughters. In my free time, she sent me to museums and on sightseeing excursions in her chauffeur-driven car. She also gave me some lovely antique jewelry as gifts. She entrusted me with shopping for some of the children's clothes, although most of them were custom made for them by the best Parisian couturiers.

From the end of June and through September, the household removed from Paris to Hendaye, on the border between France and Spain, where the countess owned an exquisite little chateau, the Chateau d'Oriole. It was built in the Spanish style and sat on a mountain, with a beautiful view over farmland and woods. There was a guesthouse on the grounds, especially built for the children. As the governess, I lived in luxurious guest quarters over the garage.

Time passed, and the children were learning fast. After about a year they spoke Dutch fluently, and I started them on German. But even though they made all the progress academically that one could wish for, I was not happy about their social isolation. I wanted them to have some contact with ordinary children, not just the select few from other aristocratic families. I discussed this with their parents and proposed that they attend a regular school at least during the months we were in Holland. The parents agreed with me, and I was told that a car and chauffeur would be at my disposition to take them back and forth to school.

But I had a different idea. I wanted them to go to school on bicycles, like almost every other Dutch schoolchild. I bought a bicycle for the older girl and taught her how to ride it. For the first few months I took the younger one on the carrier seat at the back of my bicycle, but soon she got a bike of her own and managed just fine. It was only about a fifteen-minute ride to a parochial school nearby. I bought the children sturdy rain capes, and off they went, rain or shine.

They liked the arrangement, and the exercise did them good. Apart from any other benefits, it also helped them perfect their Dutch, since that was the only language spoken in school. It also made it easier for me to keep up with the official school curriculum and to make sure they did not fall behind in anything while we were traveling. On the whole they were way ahead of the other children, especially in general knowledge.

War clouds started to gather over Europe. We were vacationing in France again when war broke out. It was the summer of 1939, and I had been with the little countesses for five years.

The countess decided to send the children to Switzerland for the duration of the war and begged me to go with them. But even though Holland was not yet at war, I did not want to leave my country in case I was needed there. So as soon as they had found a replacement for me, I said goodbye to my former charges, and thus my life among the aristocracy ended. Years later, I happened to meet the count at a cocktail party, and he expressed his appreciation for what I had done for his daughters.

In following Jeanne through the adventures of her earliest professional engagements, it is remarkable to see how the methods she eventually employed with such success at Linwood were basically already part of her arsenal at that time. Together with the philosophy that guided her educational approach they are all reflected in the vignettes offered in this chapter.

Most basically, she made no distinction in how she treated people based on their station in life, but had a deep respect for the humanity we all share. Aristocrat or ambassador, pimp or petty thief, she approached them all from the assumption that they were doing the best they could and that they were deserving of help if they were in need.

While she had deep faith, she resisted dogma and was never bound by rigid social conventions. She accepted the need for them as well as for the rules that define societal interactions, but she challenged or broke them without hesitation when she felt that it was necessary to set things to rights.

All of her life Jeanne Simons displayed extraordinary courage and persistence when it came to addressing and solving problems and overcoming obstacles related to the welfare of others: children in her care, desperate parents, her country, and her family. She was also undaunted by challenges to her own physical survival and pursued any goal she set herself with ingenuity and single-minded determination.

But that which most prominently defined the success of her teaching and treatment method were innate qualities she possessed, refined by her training. We talk about "born teachers." Jeanne was a born healer. Among the components of her treatment arsenal that she was able to verbalize were some she seemed to know instinctively:

> She was convinced that engaging in a power struggle with a child is not only futile but destroys the trust that allows a child to participate in educational moments.
>
> She was infinitely patient but keenly observant and thus ready to seize the "teachable moment" when an intervention could be successful.
>
> Most importantly, she always looked for something meaningful to the child that could be used as a motivator, like Christine's imaginary "husband" and later, with autistic children, compulsions or obsessions. Rather than trying to extinguish "bad behavior" by punishment, she accepted it and used it to get past the child's defenses. Her motto was then, and remained throughout her career, that successful teaching and therapy is based on "walking behind the child," the better to observe and guide him.

While she denied for a long time that intuition had anything to do with her almost magical touch with children on the autism spectrum, she later came to understand that something in these children called out to her and that her own experiences as an individual with autism may have helped her to gain access to them.

Exile, 1940

7

I had gone from rags to riches in my previous two jobs and had discovered that it was no easier to adjust to life among the very wealthy than to the hardships at St. Vincentius. Each brought its own difficulties and rewards. And in each, I learned and experienced a lot that came in useful at some later time. Now my life was about to take another unexpected turn.

It became ever more likely that Holland would be invaded by the Germans. But many people still believed that we would not become involved. Holland had been at peace since 1813. Even the most pessimistic people could not openly admit that it was just a matter of time before we, too, would be drawn into this war. As the weeks went by, Holland started to prepare for the worst. Shelters were built, barricades put up, and people hid their valuables and started to hoard food. But everyone stayed calm, still not believing that an invasion was near.

The Red Cross became active. Along with many other young women, I signed up for one of their courses in first aid. After several weeks of learning the basic procedures, a group of us was asked to continue with more advanced training. In case of fighting, trained aides would be needed on the battlefields to help stabilize the wounded before they could be taken to the field hospitals.

The training was very intense and covered a lot of ground in a short time. We learned things nurses are not usually taught until their last year in nursing school and even then would only be allowed to perform in an emergency, if no doctor was available.

As part of our training we were assigned to both day and night shifts in regular hospitals, which included a three-week rotation on a ward for incurable and terminally ill patients. We were also given a quick course in recognizing hysterical reactions and how to distinguish them from true battle fatigue and emotional trauma. Anyone who panicked at the sight of blood was dismissed. I seem to remember that you were allowed one fainting spell but were not given a second chance. Eventually we were put on night duty on our own. During my first stint, one patient developed an embolism in her leg. Another had a heart attack. Only when I had administered emergency aid did I call the head nurse.

Following six months of intensive training we had three days of examinations, both written and oral. Those who passed were given a secret code by which they could be mobilized quickly, in case of war. The codes also told each person where they would be deployed. We had agreed among ourselves that those who were not married and had no dependents would ask to be given the most dangerous assignments. This arrangement was accepted by the people in charge, and my assignment was to have been the airfield in Rotterdam. As I heard later, this was one of the first places that was bombed, with heavy loss of life and few survivors. But by that time I was no longer in Holland, and this probably saved my life.

I had apparently done so well in the exams that I was asked whether I would like to continue training to become a registered nurse. But even though I liked the work, I was not sure that it was what I wanted to do with my life. I asked for some time to think it over. While I was still mulling over the idea of whether I should enter nursing school, I received a phone call from the American ambassador to Holland, who had apparently heard about me through my previous employers. He asked me whether I would be willing to take on a brief assignment.

His seven-year-old daughter, Audrey, was attending school in Switzerland. She had been accompanied by her governess who was supposed to keep an eye on her, even though Audrey was a boarder at the school. There had been some problem, and the woman had to be dismissed. This meant that now the little girl was stranded in Switzerland. The ambassador wanted me to travel there and bring her back.

I knew Audrey. She was one of the children with whom the little countesses had been allowed to socialize. She had always struck me as a sad child, overprotected and precocious. She rarely smiled and looked more like a little old woman than like a young girl. I sympathized with the parents' plight. Nevertheless, I refused the assignment. I had barely made it back from France and did not want to risk leaving Holland again. By now it was March of 1940 and the invasion of Holland seemed only a matter of time. I did not want to be away from home, where I would be needed.

A few days after my initial refusal, the ambassador and his wife came to my home. They were middle-aged people and seemed too old to be the parents of a young child. They pleaded with me to reconsider. Audrey's mother was in poor health and did not want to leave her husband. They knew that I had held a position of great responsibility in the count's family, and they felt they could trust me. They were frantic and very persuasive. I was only going to be gone a few days, at most a week, and would be well paid. I would also carry diplomatic papers to assure safe passage. Still I hesitated.

I was engaged. Because of a motorcycle accident, my fiancé had a slight limp and had not been called up for army service, unlike my brothers and most of the young men of our generation. We had plans for a June wedding. I told my fiancé about the ambassador's request and about my reservations. He was very tenderhearted and wondered out loud how we would feel if it was our own child stranded somewhere by herself. This tipped the scales, and I accepted the assignment. However, I made it very clear that I was doing this as a favor. I did not want to be paid except for having my expenses reimbursed and wanted no further responsibility for the child once we were back.

It was April of 1940 when I left on my mission. I carried a letter, signed by Audrey's parents, giving me full power of attorney while she was in my charge. I also had carte blanche as far as money was concerned, with access to a Swiss bank account. Just in case, I had asked for the names of the family's American lawyer and banker and for a list of other contacts in the United States. The lawyer was to be notified of the fact that Audrey was no longer in the care of her previous governess. I also suggested that the American consul in Switzerland be alerted to my arrival and assignment. I did not foresee any particular problems, but I wanted to be sure that there were people I could turn to in case anything should happen to Audrey's parents.

Before I left, I made the parents promise that they would notify me immediately if it looked as if war was imminent. I made it very clear to them that if Holland was in danger and they wanted their child to stay in Switzerland, they would have to make other arrangements for her. I was not going to be responsible for her, but would return forthwith to Holland. They assured me that every eventuality had been taken care of. Still I had an uncomfortable feeling about the whole enterprise and wanted to make as sure as possible that Audrey would be taken care of, no matter what happened.

I traveled to Lausanne, in Switzerland, and from there to Gstaad, a little mountain village where Audrey's school was located. As soon as I saw her, I knew that she was both frightened and ill. She seemed scared of the school itself, the slopes—where she had been expected to learn to ski—and even the hotel where her governess had been staying. I decided to remove her from the whole environment and called her parents to tell them that we would temporarily move to another village, which I knew from my time with the little countesses. It was closer to Lausanne, where I knew a good pediatrician.

I wanted to make sure that Audrey was well enough to travel. I did not like her extreme thinness. Her skin had a yellow tinge and she had a slight fever. The parents approved my plans. They wanted me to stay in some fancy hotel, but I preferred to rent rooms in the chalet where I used to lodge during previous vacations. I felt that it would be easier to get the proper diet for her in a private setting. The owners were wonderful people and happy to accommodate us. The doctor came and confirmed what I had suspected. Audrey had hepatitis and could not travel.

I have no idea why her condition had not been recognized at her boarding school. She was so weak that she could hardly walk. She was unable to keep food down and was losing weight rapidly. When I bathed her, it was like handling a little skeleton. The doctor insisted that she could not afford to lose any more weight and instructed me to feed her a teaspoon of sugar water every fifteen minutes. Once that stayed down, I was to increase it to a tablespoon. This had to be done around the clock, and after a few days Audrey was able to keep down small quantities of solids from the diet prescribed for her. Slowly, she got stronger.

The news about the war was very disquieting. From what I could gather, the Germans had already penetrated deeply into France. The famed Maginot Line, which was thought to be impregnable, had fallen. In fact, the Germans had simply gone around it. I decided to move to Lausanne where it was easier to keep in touch with Holland by phone.

It was now the end of April. French refugees poured into Switzerland. They came by train, by car, and on foot. Lausanne resembled a madhouse. I kept calling Audrey's family, and they kept promising that they were making travel arrangements for us.

On the ninth of May, I finally got the message that I could leave for Paris the following day and from there proceed to Holland. Neither the United States nor the Netherlands had entered the war as yet, and my diplomatic papers should see us through without difficulties. I quickly packed. Early the next morning, the hotel manager came to my room and told me that Holland had been invaded during the night.

I tried to call Holland, but without success. I called the Dutch consul in Bern, but he too had no way of getting through. I called the State Department in Washington. They had no precise information to give me. Holland seemed to have been sealed off hermetically.

One of the things that has always been hardest for me is to be in a state of limbo. If I do not know what comes next, I cannot guard against any feelings that might threaten me. I felt trapped and helpless. To avoid becoming overpowered by panic, I stopped myself from feeling anything. I became icily calm.

I called the lawyer in New York. He thought that the best thing was to try to get Audrey to the States. I was not ready for this. I was sure that I would be able to make it back to Holland somehow, if I did not have to worry about Audrey, but I also knew that I could not afford to waste energy on such thoughts. When it came right down to it, I really had no choice. The child was my responsibility until I could hand her over to her parents or one of their representatives. I would have to take it one day at a time and think of nothing but the next necessary step.

I waited and waited. The Dutch consulate in Bern knew no more than anyone else. The invasion had been sudden, and all communications were disrupted. The consul told me that he planned to send his own family to America and advised me to take Audrey there also. He would let me know when a group left, so I would not have to travel alone. While in Lausanne, I had met several friends of Audrey's parents. When they heard about my plan to take her to America, they gave me all sorts of dire warnings. Wealthy children, they told me, were vulnerable to being kidnapped. I must never let her out of my sight. Any place other than Park Avenue, Fifth Avenue, and Lexington Avenue was unsafe. If I set foot outside those boundaries, I was likely to get robbed. I listened politely but didn't worry about what I heard. I had other things on my mind.

It is difficult to describe the atmosphere in Switzerland at that time. In addition to the French refugees, there was also an influx of Germans, mostly Jewish people, who told about the prosecution of the Jewish population by the Nazis. I was told that Jewish refugee groups had been infiltrated by German spies and was warned to be careful about who I talked to. I could not imagine why a spy should want to talk to me in the first place, but it was all part of the confusion and the paranoia of the time.

Toward the end of May, I again called the consul in Bern. It turned out that he had indeed sent his children to the States but had forgotten about us. Then the lawyer called me from New York, telling me that an American ship, the SS *Manhattan*, would be leaving for the States from Italy sometimes during the first week of June. He told me to get myself to Genoa as quickly as possible, where I would find two first-class tickets waiting for me. At last, I had something to go by.

I was told that every passenger could only bring one suitcase. I packed warm clothes for Audrey, took the bare minimum for myself, and gave the rest of our things to the Red Cross for the refugees. Then we took the train to Genoa. It was full, but we had seats for the whole trip and got to our destination sometime during the night. Since boarding was to start in the morning, we spent the rest of the night sitting on our luggage on the pier. I tried to keep poor little Audrey as comfortable as possible.

There was utter chaos on the dock where the SS *Manhattan* was berthed. It was crowded with people, rich and poor, with and without tickets, all of them desperate to get away. There was a police cordon to keep unauthorized people from getting on board. Anxiety among those waiting for passage rose to an even higher pitch when they saw the *Rex*, an Italian luxury liner, leave port. The ship carried no passengers, and the rumor spread that Italy would soon enter the war.

Finally, they started to "process" the passengers. When it was our turn, I was told that Audrey would be allowed to go, because she was American, but that I did not qualify, despite my diplomatic papers. It was too late to make other arrangements for Audrey, and I could not possibly let her travel alone. I insisted that either both of us went, or she would have to stay behind also. Because she was the child of an American ambassador they obviously felt some obligation to assure her safety, so they ended up allowing me on board. Italy entered the war two days after we sailed.

The ship carried more than twice the number of passengers it was designed to handle. There must have been close to twenty-five hundred people on board, many of whom were crowded together on deck. Theoretically we had first-class passages booked. But we ended up sharing our cabin with four other people. There were not enough lifeboats, and

I was given one life belt for the two of us. Despite the overcrowding, food did not appear to be a problem. Everything was handled beautifully and went very smoothly.

I remember standing on deck as we were sailing toward the Strait of Gibraltar. Slowly we passed these last outposts of Europe, then headed out to sea. The land I could see got smaller and smaller, then it disappeared altogether.

I was aware that one of my handicaps was going to be that I did not know English. I listened to the Americans talk, and wherever I went I carried a small dictionary with me, which I studied from the first to the last page. I had also bought a small phrase book. I never let on that I spoke Dutch, German, or French, or even that I could understand these languages. I tried to say everything in English, from asking what time it was to ordering something to eat. This way, I hoped to become independent as soon as possible.

At last we arrived in New York. I saw the Statue of Liberty, standing there to welcome us to the land of freedom. Everyone was on deck to greet the great lady. People sang, cried, and hugged each other. They were relieved to be safe. I had left behind a country full of suffering and agony I could barely imagine, a country where I wanted to be with all my heart to help in any way possible. I looked at Audrey and hoped that she would never realize the price I was paying for her safety.

It was a rainy, cold afternoon when we docked. Hundreds of people crowded the dock, carrying flowers or waving flags. They were speaking every imaginable language. I stood in that crowd for a long time. I had been told that the lawyer would meet us. It took hours, but we finally cleared customs, and the lawyer accompanied me to the beautiful hotel where he had booked rooms for us. I think it was The Pierre, on Central Park. In any case, it was very fancy, and we had a beautiful suite on one of the upper floors. I remember a huge bedroom, all decorated in silver and black, with a big mirror. I sat on the windowsill, stunned by the incredible view. There were thousands of lights, with endless columns of cars moving like a bright snake down the avenues. Did anyone here know what a blackout was? Driving down the broad avenues, did anyone think of the thousands of refugees walking for days with their few possessions to find a country not yet at war?

I looked at the wonderful sight from my hotel room and did not feel anything. I knew that I would store the experience away and maybe, at some later time, I could recall it and get some benefit from it. For now, I could not take it in. At last, I went to bed to spend a sleepless night, waiting for the new day, for a new beginning, in a country I did not want to be in, with a responsibility that weighed almost more than I could carry.

Managing emotions is something most people with autism cannot do effectively, which is why children with the disorder often have temper outbursts of epic proportions. Jeanne Simons is unusual in that she was able to develop strategies to deal with emotions, either by sealing herself off from them completely or by finding an alternative to keep them from overwhelming her.

Stranded in America, 1940–1945   *8*

The year that followed was one of the most devastating of my life. I was living in limbo, and there was no way to escape. It was impossible to find out what was really happening in Europe. I had been cut off completely from anything that was familiar, and the cut had come suddenly, without warning, without a chance to brace myself.

The day after our arrival in New York, I asked for a conference with the lawyer. He had been expecting someone who spoke no English and was surprised by how much I had already picked up. I presented him with a stack of receipts for money I had spent in Switzerland and during our journey. He sent his secretary with me to buy clothes for Audrey and told me to outfit myself, too. I did not feel comfortable having money spent on me, so I bought the bare minimum.

Before we could make further plans, Audrey became ill again, this time with pneumonia. The lawyer offered to hire a nurse to take care of her, but I refused. A doctor came every day and told me what to do. By the time she was well again, I was worn out. To give me a break, the lawyer sent his secretary to the hotel and told me to take the day off.

It is difficult to explain how I felt. My whole life I had been able to face difficult situations by becoming stiff and by keeping emotions at a distance, both my own and those of others. But now I had the same kind of feeling that I had had as a small baby, that something in me was going to blow up, and if it did, the pieces might never come together again.

I had long ago decided not to cry and thought I had forgotten how, yet I felt as if, inside, I was drowning in a flood of tears. Waves of tears were pounding at me, trying to force their way out. I had to cry. But I was afraid that once I started, I might never be able to stop again. An idea struck me. I set the alarm clock for five minutes; then I went to bed and let the tears come. I stuffed the sheet in my mouth so nobody would hear me, and I sobbed and sobbed. The alarm clock went off but I couldn't stop. I gave myself another five minutes. This time when the alarm went off, I managed to stop. Some of the pressure had eased. I also knew, now, that it was safe to cry, as long as I set myself some limits. I did this a few more times over the next weeks, and then I seemed to have no tears left.

THE LAWYER THOUGHT it would be better to move Audrey out of New York. Her parents belonged to a country club outside the city that he booked us into for the rest of the summer. We returned to New York in early fall, again lodging in a hotel. The lawyer had managed to get word to Audrey's parents to let them know that she was safe. He told me they had been frantic about us. They had apparently been told that we were somewhere in France but of course had been unable to trace us. Finally, in October, word came from Holland that all American diplomats would be returning to the States. We went to meet the ship. It was a happy reunion for Audrey and her parents. I asked them about my family and was told that there was a letter from them somewhere in their luggage that they would give to me at the hotel.

They had taken suites at the Ambassador Hotel on Park Avenue, and as soon as they were settled in, the ambassador ordered up champagne to celebrate the family's reunion. A waiter handed around the champagne. There was one glass of orange juice on the tray, which he handed to Audrey. The ambassador stopped him and said: "This is for Mademoiselle." The butler gave me the orange juice and proceeded to serve champagne to the family, including Audrey. I stood frozen in disbelief at this shabby treatment. I do not know what happened to me. I did the only thing that came to mind. I simply dropped the glass and without a word I left the room. Before the door closed behind me, I heard the wife of the ambassador ask: "Why is Mademoiselle so upset?"

I waited to be given my letter from home. Dinner passed. I put Audrey to bed, and still I waited. When her mother was about to retire for the night, I finally asked for my letter. She waved me away, saying that she was too tired to look for it and would give it to me in the morning. Then she started to close the door. I could not believe what was happening. I cannot remember feeling anger. There was just utter disbelief and confusion. I stood there with my foot in the door and insisted, very politely, that I would like to have the letter—*now*. I got it. In the event, it gave me little news. There were mostly expressions of relief that I was safe. They had been worried when no one knew where I was. They hoped I would be home soon.

I cannot remember Audrey's family asking me how I had managed the whole time on my own. Nor did they ever really thank me. I had not expected thanks, but I did expect to be treated with respect. Instead, I suddenly seemed to be a nobody, nothing more than a servant.

I asked how soon they could make arrangements for my return to Holland. They thought that I was out of my mind. Didn't I know how lucky I was to be out of Europe and safely in the States? I reminded them of their promise. The ambassador became furious. He told me that he had more important things to do than to negotiate with the German Embassy on my behalf. Yet, I knew that he had had at least one meeting with high German officials to arrange for his wife's personal maid, who was German, to come to the States.

I quietly but firmly told him that if he could negotiate with the Germans on his wife's maid's behalf, he surely could do so for someone who had brought his child to safety. Again, I reminded him of his promise. He blew up at me and slammed the door in my face. I stood there feeling as if I was going to break apart, but outwardly I stayed calm. Though he literally turned purple in the face every time I touched on the subject, I persisted. He finally gave in and spoke to some German officials to see what could be done.

In the meantime, I had contacted the Dutch Embassy to find out what they knew about possible ways of returning to Holland. They told me that the only way to do this was to get permission from the Germans. Apparently the Dutch government in exile had given permission for Dutch citizens wanting to return to Holland to travel on a German visa. I got the necessary papers from Audrey's father and took them to the German Embassy. The first thing I saw, when I entered the building, was a life-size portrait of Hitler. Swastikas were displayed all over the place. I pretended that I did not know any German. I was handed from one official to another, all very polite, clicking their heels, and eventually I did get some papers.

But that was only the beginning of a series of frustrating delays. It seemed that there was always some other thing missing until, finally, I was told that I would need to get a Portuguese transit visa before I could get permission to reenter Holland. After a lot of running around and delays, I got that too. Before taking it to the Germans, I checked in again with the Dutch Embassy. There I was told that just two weeks earlier, the Dutch government had rescinded permission for Dutch citizens to travel on a German visa, and that anybody who had one would be treated as a traitor.

This news hit me like a bolt of lightning. It ended all hope of returning home while the war was going on. Up to then, I had been sustained by my single-minded determination to return to Holland. This was now no longer an option, and everything around me seemed to have collapsed. For a few days I walked around in a daze and at times wondered whether I was going to have a breakdown. But at least I was now out of the "in-between" state that had been so difficult for me. While ambiguity is a great threat to me, I am usually able to cope once I am faced with facts, however painful. Now, my situation was clear. For the time being I would have to stay in America and make the best of it. Still, it was not easy to accept this. Not only had I been abruptly severed from my own world, but my present circumstances were anything but pleasant.

AUDREY'S PARENTS SEEMED to take it for granted that I would be staying on with them and continue to look after Audrey. Months had passed, the family had moved to Washington, but a salary had never been mentioned. Nor had I been given any pocket money, although the expenses I incurred to travel to New York for my visa had been paid. When I finally brought up the subject, they quoted me a sum that was barely a third of the salary generally paid a governess in the States. I did not know any better and accepted without question, glad to have some money of my own again. Later, a friend told me that I was being taken advantage of, but I didn't really care. I was not going to get into an argument over money.

I tried to give Audrey as much of a normal life as possible. She had no dolls. I bought them for her. We played house with them and made them clothes. I took her out as often as I could. I made friends with some very nice nurses and governesses of children who belonged to the same social circle as her family. They were all amazed that I stayed with these unpleasant people. But I didn't think that I had any choice.

SOON AFTER I KNEW that I would not be returning to Holland in the foreseeable future, I began to think more seriously about Audrey's education. I had been giving her lessons ever since she had been in my charge, but I thought she should go to school. My English certainly wasn't good enough to provide her with a proper American education. I also felt that she ought to have the opportunity to associate with other children her age and lead a more normal existence. The parents agreed, and Audrey was enrolled in a fancy private school. I took her there every morning and collected her again in the afternoon. We were driven both ways by the family chauffeur in the ambassador's limousine.

Since she was in school much of the day and I had nothing to do during that time, I decided to offer my services to the Red Cross. I helped to make bandages, translated letters coming from Holland,

and generally tried to make myself useful in every possible way. Through this volunteer job I met some people from the Dutch Embassy and made friends with them. But when Audrey's parents discovered what I was doing, they became very angry. Her father told me that he expected me to stay home, in case Audrey became ill at school and had to be fetched home. I was not to leave the house. Though I felt like a caged animal, I couldn't disobey. He was my employer, after all, and I was totally dependent on him, or so I thought.

Soon after Christmas, there was a flu epidemic. Everyone recovered relatively quickly, but I developed a very high fever. A doctor was called. He was a very kind man. He told me to stay in bed and to come see him at his office the next day. I went, although my temperature was still 104 degrees. It so happened that the wife of the Dutch naval attaché had accompanied her son to the doctor's office for a checkup that same day. The doctor told her that he had just seen a very sick young Dutch woman he was worried about. He told me later that he was not only concerned about my physical illness but also not sure how I was going to survive emotionally in the family I was with. In any case, the wife of the attaché came to see me.

She knew Audrey's parents from parties. After several visits, she proposed that I come and stay with her for a while, once I was allowed to leave the bed. She seemed to be a genuinely warmhearted woman and I could not imagine anything more welcome. Somehow she got the family's permission. Two weeks later I was able to get up, and I and went to spend my convalescence with the attaché's family. The whole time I had been in bed, a very nice maid had looked after me. Neither of Audrey's parents ever came to see me.

The two weeks with this family were wonderful. They had a son and a daughter, and the whole family loved music. Every night, after dinner, they put on some classical music. But while I felt very comfortable with them, I was still anything but well. The fever had gone, but I suffered from terrific headaches, dizziness, and double vision. It was with a heavy heart that I returned to my golden cage, even though my new friends promised to stay in touch.

The doctor was clearly worried about my condition and sent me to a neurologist for a consult. He promptly hospitalized me. I think he suspected a tumor, but they did all possible neurological tests and didn't find anything. Audrey's parents were notified. The ambassador came to see me the next day. He handed me some tulips and then quickly left again. The next day, he and his family went away on vacation. They had hired a temporary nurse and taken Audrey with them. They hadn't bothered telling anyone about my hospitalization, so the whole two weeks I was there, I had no visitors. That didn't really bother me too much. I was only grateful that my family did not know about my illness, so they did not have to worry.

After I had encephalitis as a young girl, the doctor had told me that I would have to avoid all undue pressure in the future. Yet for months now I had felt like a pressure cooker without a safety valve. No wonder my poor brain revolted. I was somewhat improved after two weeks, though still far from well. My employers had returned from their trip. They knew when I was to be released from the hospital, but nobody came to pick me up and I had to take a taxi.

The weeks passed. I continued to have headaches and did not feel well. In the spring of 1941, the whole family spent a few weeks in Hot Springs, Virginia. It was a beautiful resort, with every imaginable comfort and entertainment, including horseback riding and swimming. Audrey and I shared a cottage with her parents. It was well appointed and very comfortable, although having to live at such close quarters with the ambassador was less than pleasant.

Back in Washington, things were no better. And with Audrey at school much of the day, I had too much time on my hands. Even though I was not doing much, I was constantly exhausted. My head hurt. It took an enormous amount of energy not to brood about my situation. The news out of Europe was spotty, and I had not had another sign of life from my family.

The summer brought some unexpected and welcome changes. Audrey was sent to a summer camp in New Hampshire and I went with her. The camp was located on a lake and was surrounded by trees, with a view of wooded mountains. The people who ran the camp were extremely nice, and the relaxed, friendly atmosphere, the camping and canoe trips, the nightly camp fires with singing and storytelling, and just being out in nature did me a lot of good. I still had the headaches, but instead of wondering how I would make it through each day, I was able to replenish some of my strength and store up some lovely memories.

The eight weeks passed only too quickly, and then it was time to return to Washington and the problems awaiting me there. My Dutch friends had urged me for some time to leave my position, but where would I go? How could I make a living? How much longer could I go on without direction?

December came around and one day, as I looked out of my window, I saw a sudden flurry of activity on the grounds of the Japanese Embassy. Two men came running out of the embassy building and locked the entry gates into the compound. Others seemed to be stoking several small bonfires. I sensed that something terrible was about to happen. I told Audrey's mother what I had observed and she called her husband at the State Department. He called back a little while later and told her that word had just come in that the Japanese had bombed Pearl Harbor. America was now at war.

FEW PEOPLE WERE NOT AFFECTED in some way by America's entry into the war. Sorrow, anxiety, and fear surrounded me. Now not only did I have to keep my own feelings at bay, I also had to prevent the emotions of those around me from crashing over me and sweeping me away. The Red Cross had put out an urgent call for volunteers. They especially needed trained nurse's aides to help out in hospitals, since many nurses and doctors had joined the armed forces. I told Audrey's parents that I would like to offer my services, even if it was only for one day a week. I also wanted to enroll in the course the Red Cross offered for certification as a nurse's aide. (I had been told that I would have to take it again, even though I had been trained in Holland.)

Again, permission was denied. I was told in no uncertain terms that I was hired to be available for Audrey. But this time, I was determined to fight. I asked my Dutch friends to intercede for me. They were no more no more successful than I had been. They were appalled by the insensitivity and rudeness they encountered. It was clear to them that I had to get away, and they offered to have me stay with them as long as I needed to.

I told Audrey's family that it was time they looked for another governess for her. I offered to stay on until they had found a suitable person. There was another explosion of fury from the ambassador, but it didn't bother me. Freedom was within my reach. It took several more months, then I moved in with the family of the Dutch naval attaché and joined the Red Cross.

While I was still looking for a regular job, I got a letter from the director of the camp in New Hampshire where Audrey and I had spent the previous summer. He wondered whether I might be interested in spending the summer with them as a paid counselor. Among their campers, there would be a number of youngsters of different nationalities, and they would like me to be in charge of a group of the older ones. Naturally, I accepted.

It was wonderful living close to nature again. The wall of misery that had almost crushed me seemed to move away to a safer distance and leave me some room to breathe. Nevertheless, the severe headaches returned, and by August they were again accompanied by double vision, and this time also by a loss of balance. I had no choice but to tell the camp director, who took me to a local hospital. There they performed a lumbar puncture. I don't know whether something went wrong with it; in any case, I started having trouble breathing and had to be given oxygen. The camp director was told that I should be taken to a larger hospital where there were better facilities for doing additional neurological tests. Until something could be arranged, I was taken back to the camp and put to bed there. I felt very sick, and the headaches reminded me of when I had encephalitis at age seventeen.

One of the campers had a father who was a doctor. When he came to visit his son, he heard about me and got in touch with a colleague of his who was a neurosurgeon in Boston. When he described my symptoms to him, he was told to get me to Boston as quickly as possible. One of the staff members drove me to the Lahey Clinic in Boston, where I was examined and hospitalized immediately. Ice bags were put around my head. They made the pain a little more bearable.

The neurosurgeon was one of the nicest men I had ever met. He was compassionate and understanding. After a week of tests and observations he came to my room. He sat on the edge of my bed, took my hand, and asked me how he could reach my family. I told him my circumstances and that there was no way to get in touch with anyone. The reason he wanted to speak to them was that he suspected I had a brain tumor. I would need to have exploratory surgery and possibly a more serious operation. When I asked him what my chances were to get well again, he was very honest with me. He put them at about fifty-fifty. I asked him to leave me alone for a while.

I felt as if a volcano was about to erupt within me. I wanted to cry to ease the pressure but could not. My long-conquered fears of being disabled, helpless, and dependent were surfacing. I kept thinking "fifty-fifty, fifty-fifty." But then, I suddenly became very calm. A quietness settled over me. I had a 50% chance of being crippled or of dying. Fear could not prevent this or change the odds. But I also had a 50% chance to survive. It was clearly a waste of time and energy to agonize over this. My lack of imagination also helped. *Dying* was only a word to me, and though there was some curiosity in me about what it would be like, it wasn't anything I had any experience with, and so I couldn't imagine it.

When the doctor came back, I told him that he could go ahead with the operation. My only worry was that I had no way of paying for it. He told me that I would eventually have to pay for the hospital stay, which I could do a little at a time, once I was well and working again, but that he was not going to charge anything for the operation.

I was to consider this his contribution to those caught up in the war. He wanted to know whether I had any friends who could donate blood for me. Several people from the camp, including the director, came down to have their blood typed. Unfortunately, none of it was compatible with mine.

When it had become evident that I was seriously ill, the camp director had called the Dutch Embassy, even though I had not wanted him to do so. I didn't want anyone to feel that they had to come all the way up from Washington to see me. But the wife of the naval attaché made the trip anyway, and also ended up as a blood donor.

The doctor came to see me again the day before the operation. Again, he sat on my bed. He had paper and pencil with him and asked whether I wouldn't like to write some letters to my family and my fiancé in case something happened to me. I thought that this was a good idea, and he left me to it. But when he came back, I handed him a blank piece of paper. The surprise on his face made me smile. I explained that since no one knew how much longer the war would last, it might be years before any letters could be delivered. If I didn't survive, my family might suffer more from getting a message from me so long after my death. If I did survive, writing the letters would have been a waste of energy on my part, which I could ill afford at this point.

What I didn't tell him was that when it came right down to it, I had not known what to write. They would have been unnecessarily hurt and confused if I had told them the truth, which was that I was glad to be alone, because this way I would not have to deal with their pain. They would not have understood, but I was unable to make up a message that was meaningful to them and that they would like.

I made the doctor promise that should I not survive, he would write to my family, telling them things that would console them in their grief. I asked him to tell them that my death had been peaceful, that I had not suffered, and that I had died surrounded by friends and like a good Christian, provided with the holy sacraments. When he promised to do this, everything became very peaceful. I had taken care of everything I had control over. Now the world full of violence and sorrow seemed far removed.

He told me that before he operated, he wanted to do one more test, another lumbar puncture. But this time, instead of tapping the spine, he was going to bore two little holes in the back of my head. This was going to be done under full anesthesia, and depending on the result, he would decide whether an operation was indeed the way to go. I asked him whether he could wake me up and tell me the results of the test, but I was told that it would not be possible. He also warned me that my head would have to be shaved. I asked him to leave a fringe of hair in the front, and he promised to see to it.

Before I was wheeled into the operating room, I made up my mind that I would speak French when I woke up. I had heard that people emerging from anesthesia often talked before they were fully conscious. My whole life, nobody had ever had access to my inner world, and I wanted to make sure that it stayed that way. And sure enough, when I was coming to, I remember speaking French.

As soon as I was fully conscious, the doctor came to assure me that all was well. What he had found was not a tumor, but adhesions from the scars of the encephalitis I had had as a girl. He had been able to remove them and had also taken a piece of bone from my left temple area to help drain some fluid that had been building up.

I was so relieved that I didn't have a tumor and could be looking forward to regaining my independence that I did not inquire too closely into the cause of my recent illness or ask after possible long-term consequences. I was out of the hospital in ten days. I had had no visitors, but arrangements had been made through friends at the embassy that I could stay in Boston for a few additional days, until I was strong enough to travel. I was still pretty weak, so I broke my trip in New York, where I stayed with friends I had made in New Hampshire. Then I returned to Washington and the Dutch family that had previously taken me in.

I quickly regained my strength. Soon the only memory of the operation was my bald head. I covered it with scarves matching my clothes.

The doctor had kept his promise, and the fringe in front helped to make me look almost normal until my hair could grow in again.

As soon as I was strong enough, I started looking for a job. In fact, this is the only time in my life that I have actively looked for work. I was lucky. The Christ Child Settlement House needed a director. I got the job and the pay was good enough so I could afford to look for a place of my own to rent. But the son of the family I had been living with had been called to duty in the Dutch army. Their daughter was getting married. Suddenly their house seemed very empty, and they told me that I would be doing them a favor if I stayed on with them. I felt very comfortable with them and accepted gratefully.

Working hours at my new job were from about three o'clock in the afternoon until nine at night. Most mornings I helped out at the Red Cross again, and part of every weekend I volunteered at Walter Reed Hospital, a military hospital where wounded soldiers were being cared for.

Through the Dutch Embassy, I now had access to news smuggled out of Holland via England. I read about friends and acquaintances who had been killed or taken prisoner, and about areas that had been bombed and destroyed. But there was still no direct news from my family. Despite all the uncertainties and the news of war disaster, I no longer felt as if I was doing a balancing act on a tightrope without a safety net. My days were filled with meaningful work, and I was living with people I liked. Volunteering at the Red Cross and at Walter Reed gave me the feeling that I was doing my part in the war.

At Walter Reed, I was assigned to the ward for the most severely wounded. It was hard to see young men spend their lives suspended between two planks, not able to do anything for themselves. Some of them, especially those with severe spinal injuries, would have to be taken care of for the rest of their lives. They had to be turned at regular intervals so they spent half of their time on their backs and half of it on their stomachs.

After a while I was asked whether I would like to work with the amputees. Most of them were in relatively good health and were learning to use artificial limbs. They were a rowdy group. The people in charge had apparently heard that I was working at a settlement house and thought that I might have the ability to keep some kind of order on the ward. Although alcoholic beverages were not allowed on the ward, there always seemed to be plenty of them around, especially after visiting hours. This was when my shift began.

I quickly established a good rapport with these soldiers. They were so young. Many of them were barely more than boys. One day when I came in, the nurse told me that they were unmanageable. There was yelling, laughing, and singing, even some fighting. They had obviously been at the liquor again. It was bedtime, and their artificial limbs had been taken off. These were placed next to each patient's bed, and some of the men were using them to take swipes at each other. When they saw me, they all started clamoring for my attention. They wanted their backs rubbed or some other service performed.

I paid no attention but quietly went around the ward, gathered up all of the artificial limbs, and put them in the far corner, away from the beds. They caught on to what I was doing and demanded that I return them. I ignored them. They asked the nurse to intercede, but she just smiled and told me to handle the situation my way. Then she left the room. I waited until everybody had calmed down. Then I told them that whenever I was on duty I would do the same thing, if there was any drinking or rowdiness. I didn't care whether it was daytime or evening. Then I gave them back their limbs. There was some confusion about which belonged to who, but we eventually got it sorted out. They didn't hold it against me, and I worked on this ward for the rest of the war. I got along well with everybody, especially the soldiers who were no worse than naughty boys and despite their past experiences a lot of fun to be with.

My work at the settlement house, on the other hand, was not easy. The previous director was about to retire. There were presently no other staff, and I had been asked to run it by myself as best I could, until another director could be found. The center was conceived as an after-school program for school-age children, and a big crowd of them were always waiting by the time the doors opened at about three o'clock in the afternoon. There was a gym where the children could play ball, and games and toys were kept in rooms on the ground floor. The second floor was only supposed to be used for meetings, and the children were not allowed upstairs.

One of the problems with the program was that there were no organized activities and not enough games available for the number of children it was supposed to serve. Also, the toys were in very poor shape and should have been replaced a long time ago. Another problem was that a number of older teenagers seemed to have infiltrated the program. After a few days, I realized that I would generally see them come in but then tended to lose track of them. I also never saw them leave with the rest of the children.

One night, after everyone had left and I was making the rounds before locking up, I thought I heard the sound of voices coming from the second floor. I went to investigate, and the mystery of the missing teenagers was solved. I found six of them in a room filled with smoke. Some of them were drinking. Others were in various stages of undress and engaged in activities one would not expect to see in public. I suspected that this kind of thing had been going on for quite a while, right under the nose of the previous director—a dedicated but somewhat naive woman who had been ready to retire for some time.

I told the group that it was past closing time and they would have to leave. They just laughed and told me to get lost, using language I did not know and was therefore not bothered by. I told them that I would wait downstairs to let them out. They didn't budge. Finally they started to drift down, but they seemed intent on a confrontation. I stood my ground, looking them straight in the eye. One of them asked in an insolent tone of voice just what I was going to do. They were a threatening group of young adults, but my adrenaline was flowing. I grabbed the biggest young man of the bunch by the collar, somehow frog-marched him to the front door, and simply threw him out.

That took the group by surprise. I asked them who wanted to be the next one thrown out. They cussed at me, but they left. I locked the door and then had to sit down. I found that I was shaking, whether from the physical effort or as a reaction to the whole scene, I do not know. Outside, a few stones were thrown, but by the time I was ready to leave, they had all gone.

THE NEXT DAY I CALLED the president of the board and told him what had happened. I requested permission to close the house for a month to have a chance to reorganize the whole program, and he gave it to me without any hesitation. I spent part of that month going around the neighborhood, making home visits and talking to parents. I wanted to know what they expected from the program and told them that I would need their cooperation to run a decent recreation center for their children. I saw a lot of different families, much poverty, but also homes with working parents who were looking for a safe place for their children while they were at work.

I had club cards printed and was able to organize some volunteers to help me develop and supervise a program. We decided to keep the center open on Saturdays and to add activities especially designed for adolescents. For example, we organized coed parties and dances for them on Saturday nights. We asked the parents to make sure that their youngsters came home promptly from these affairs, which usually ended around midnight.

Once the program was running smoothly, the Christ Child Settlement House board hired a new director, which left me more time to explore additional ways in which the center could serve the neighborhood. We started a supper club, for example, where children could learn to cook and get a decent meal. Later, I involved the welfare mothers and taught them how to plan and cook inexpensive, nourishing meals and even helped them work out a budget.

THINGS WERE GOING BETTER for me now. Between this job and my volunteering at the Red Cross and at Walter Reed, I was kept busy and felt that I was doing useful work. I continued to live with the Dutch couple and had a nice circle of friends. It all helped me to keep the thoughts about the war, Holland, and the future under control. But after about a year, I began to have kidney trouble. Again, I had to go to the hospital.

Exploratory surgery revealed that I had something called a "pancake kidney," probably a congenital defect. The doctor thought that the kidney was still functional and could be saved. But after a few days I developed a high fever, obviously caused by an infection. Despite every effort to combat it, I got weaker and weaker. I was put on the critically ill list and even was administered the last rites. I was too sick to know what was happening, but I pulled through. When I was a little better again, the doctor told me, the kidney had to come out. They operated as soon as I was strong enough.

Recovery took a long time. I was in the hospital for about six weeks before I was allowed to return to my Dutch friends to recuperate. Luckily, the Dutch Embassy had a fund from which assistance was provided for Dutch nationals stranded in the United States who were taken ill, so my hospital expenses were taken care of.

I didn't need much money for myself, but every time I received a paycheck I went shopping. I wanted to be prepared for the end of the war, when it would be possible for me to return to Holland. I bought anything I thought might be lacking in a war-ravaged country: warm clothes, underwear, knitting wool, and shoes, dry goods and canned foods, and any other imaginable necessity.

By 1944 it was possible to start sending care packages through the Red Cross. The packages had to be a prescribed size and weight and wrapped in the right kind of wrapping material. From my storeroom full of things I had accumulated by then, I sent as many packages as were accepted. I filled any little space between larger items with tissues, thread, needles, and safety pins. We had heard that the stores in Holland were completely empty and that before they withdrew, the Germans had looted and removed everything that wasn't nailed down.

When I had been working at the settlement house for almost three years, the end of the war was becoming more of a reality. I begged the Dutch Embassy to get me a passage back to Holland at the earliest possible moment. I was supervising a summer camp for girls, organized by the settlement house, when the armistice was declared. For the few days leading up to it, everyone had their radios on night and day. As soon as we heard the news, we went to the chapel, where we held a thanksgiving ceremony. Then we all went down to the water, carrying candles, and made a big bonfire.

Sometime earlier I had received a message through the Red Cross that everyone in my family was alive, although two of my brothers had been deported to work camps in Germany and my family had been evacuated from their home in Scheveningen, which was then occupied by German soldiers. It was the first direct news I had had in almost five years; it had taken a good six months to reach me, however, so it didn't do too much to reassure me. Also, I had denied myself all feelings for so long that the news did not seem to touch me one way or another. I was emotionally empty, equally incapable of joy for the survivors as of sorrow for lost friends. But the urge to get back to Holland was as strong as ever.

Finally, I got word that passage had been secured for me on the first ship carrying civilians. It was a battered old troopship, leaving for Europe to bring home American soldiers. My friends drove me to New York. I had thirteen pieces of luggage—suitcases and crates full of the goods I had assembled over the previous three years. The ship passed the Statue of Liberty and with it I left behind five years of my life that had been unusually difficult and yet also rewarding and interesting in many ways.

Early readers wondered why Jeanne feared that a brain tumor might leave her disabled, since as a person with autism she was clearly disabled already. At this point in her life, Jeanne had not yet realized that she was living with autism. Even once she did, she never thought of herself as disabled, since she was strong in body and mind and had always been able to do anything she set her mind on. What she was afraid of was to become disabled in a way that would make her physically dependent on the care of others. And as we have seen, during several serious illnesses she put every ounce of her formidable determination into overcoming any physical disability that would limit her independence.

It may also strike some readers as odd that Jeanne was concerned about having a shaved head, since such vanity appears totally alien to the seeming disregard she showed for her own person all along. She told me, for example, that when coming upon her reflection in a mirror unexpectedly, she would not recognize herself. While I never directly addressed this seeming incongruity with her, I think that the "disguise" of a fringe of hair under a headscarf stemmed from her urgent desire to avoid notice and, what would be worse, pity, since the emotions of others were much more difficult for her to deal with than her own.

Jeanne's work at the Christ Child Settlement House brought her in contact with its founder, Mary Merrick, who as a young woman had founded the National Christ Child Society, set up as a Catholic charity organization to serve impoverished children. The settlement house was one of many organizations funded by the society. Through her work at the settlement house, Jeanne joined the organization and became friends with the elderly Miss Merrick, who had lived at Linwood, in Ellicott City, with her family as a young girl. Although the house was later sold to the family from whom Jeanne acquired it, it seems too much of a coincidence that Jeanne just happened to buy this particular house without being aware of its connection to her friend.

Readers who are interested in the fascinating history of Linwood, going back to the 1780s and including the remarkable Mary Merrick, are referred to the history section of Linwood Center's website (at www.linwoodcenter.org/about/history/), where they can access the chapter "Linwood," by Celia M. Holland, from her book *Ellicott City, Maryland: Milltown USA,* and a 2012 *Baltimore Sun* article, "Howard County's Uncanonized Saint, Mary Merrick of Linwood."

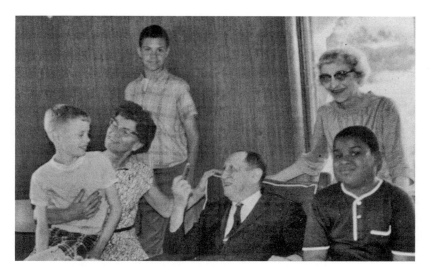

Jeanne Simons along with Dr. Leo Kanner, Miss Becky—a staffer—
and young residents of the Linwood School, Ellicott City, Maryland.
Courtesy of the Linwood Center.

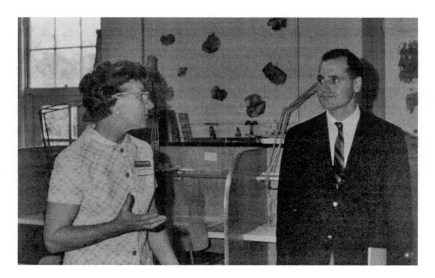

Jeanne Simons conversing with Charles B. Ferster at the Linwood
School, Ellicott City, Maryland, 1966. Ferster, a behavioral psychologist
and pioneer in the field of applied behavior analysis, was working with
Jeanne on a research project at Linwood. Courtesy of the Linwood Center.

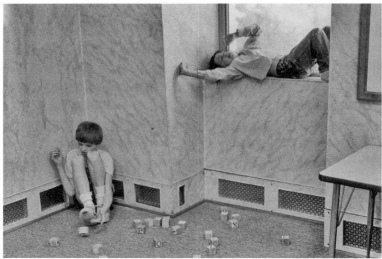

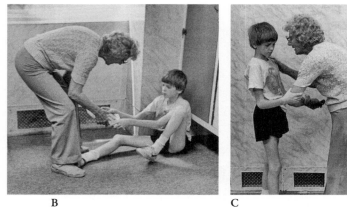

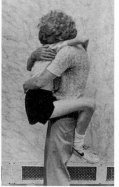

A

B   C   D

Sequence showing Jeanne's method of interacting with children diagnosed with autism spectrum disorder at Linwood School, Ellicott City, Maryland: **A**, Observation of behavior; **B**, Initial conversation and intervention; **C**, Reassurance and reinforcement; **D**, Connection. From *The Hidden Child*; courtesy of Woodbine House publishers.

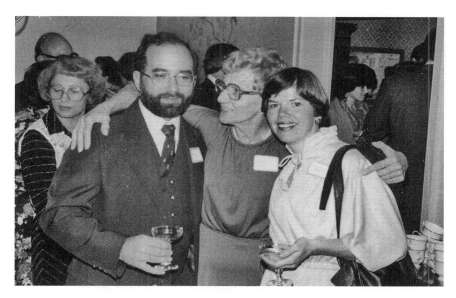

Jeanne Simons along with two graduates from the Linwood School,
Ellicott City, Maryland. Courtesy of the Linwood Center.

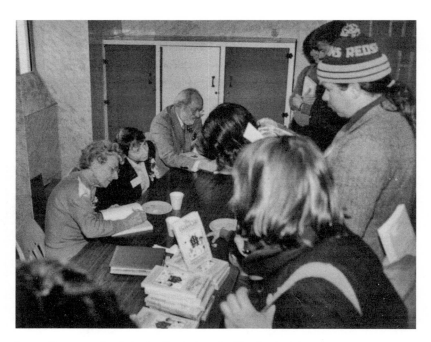

Jeanne Simons at a book signing for the launch of her book with
Sabine Oishi, *The Hidden Child: The Linwood Method for Reaching
the Autistic Child*, 1987.

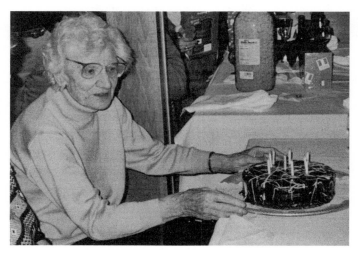

Jeanne Simons celebrating her ninetieth birthday in 1999.
Courtesy of the Linwood Center.

Back in Holland, 1945–1947 9

The trip to Holland was very rough. We ran into a hurricane and just about everybody was seasick. I love the sea and enjoy stormy weather, so it did not affect me. What was much more difficult to withstand were the emotional storms that swept the ship. Most of the passengers had been separated from their families for the duration of the war. Nobody had any idea of what they would find after years of fighting and devastation. The closer we got to Europe, the more intense the emotions became. People were drinking to quiet their fear, many were crying, some became hysterical. I had little contact with the rest of the passengers. I had to protect myself against their emotions and also prepare for the reunion with my family and friends, which would naturally be highly charged. Once again, I withdrew far into myself. I became unfeeling, as if I were made out of stone. I heard what was being said to me, but it had no real meaning. I looked but did not see. Alone, behind my impenetrable wall, I was temporarily at peace.

When I finally arrived home, I found that my family had miraculously survived intact and relatively unscathed. My brothers returned unharmed from the labor camp in Germany, and thanks to my food packages everybody was relatively strong and healthy. After their home had been taken over by the Germans, they had been lucky enough to find another one not too far away from the old neighborhood.

My fiancé, who had not been in the army, had also survived and seemed to be doing well. In fact, I had the uncomfortable feeling that he was doing too well. I wondered how he had come through the occupation so seemingly untouched by the hardships everyone else had suffered. Nothing was ever said, but by tacit mutual consent our engagement became a thing of the past.

All through the reunion with my family and friends I remained calm and unmoved. I listened to their stories of horror and hardship, looked at the devastation all around me, and nothing within me stirred. They all had so much to tell, so much to unburden themselves of, that they never probed how I had gotten through these past years. I was grateful for that. All they saw in me was the one who had been spared, who had been safe while they lived through the terrors of the war. They were thankful that I had been in a position to alleviate their suffering and that my packages had helped stave off the cold and starvation over the past two years.

Even now, it is difficult for me to think about those first few weeks back in Holland. Everything I had known and held on to through the years of my exile was gone. Not just people, but the land itself was changed. We now lived in a different house. The old one had been close to the shore, and the whole area had been cleared of buildings by the Germans. They had also destroyed the beautiful woods near our old home, which had been my childhood refuge. I have always loved trees. They have been my most comforting friends. There had been a lot of very old trees in these woods. The Germans had destroyed them all, chopping down every last tree for miles around.

As time went on, I became alarmed at my continued state of unfeelingness. It was safe, but it was also dangerous. It reminded me of the time I had realized how easy it would be to stay in hiding under my uncle's dining room table forever. If I wanted to go on living I had to participate in life somehow, and that included being in touch with my feelings. The trick was to allow myself to feel without being totally overwhelmed and destroyed.

As so often before, I turned to nature for help. I took a walk through the devastated woods, touching the stumps of the mutilated trees. Slowly, the feelings I had held at bay throughout my years in exile and during my return home came back to me. At last, I could acknowledge the loss, the grief, the anger, and the relief I had closed off. I was no longer a stone but a hurting, living being, among other living things that had been hurt. And I could weep for my pain, because the friends around me did not respond to my tears. With them I was safe.

What I had to accept was that I had become a stranger in my own country, which was no longer the country I remembered. Nor was I the same person who had left here five years earlier. Much had happened to me. I had twice come close to death, found rewarding work, made new friends, and seen and learned a lot, while Holland had undergone the devastations of the war. Friends and acquaintances had been deported and killed, wounded and maimed. They had frozen and starved and had lost homes, jobs, health, and loved ones. The face of the country had been totally changed through heavy bombardments, and its economy was devastated by five years of occupation. Poverty was everywhere. Most people lived barely above the subsistence level. Many only survived by engaging in criminal activities, such as black marketeering.

There was a serious shortage of food and clothing. Many houses had been destroyed and most of the ones still standing had windows missing. Since no glass was available, the openings were covered with paper and cardboard. Many people lived in damaged buildings and under overcrowded conditions. There was clearly a lot of work to be done before their lives could return to even a semblance of normality. For myself, I did not think about the needs of the present. My only question was where I might be the most useful.

Some of the American diplomats I had met through my friends at the Dutch Embassy in Washington came to Holland as members of the American Embassy. I was glad to see them, especially the newly appointed American naval attaché and his wife and little girl. They were warm, compassionate, and generous people, and they wanted to do something constructive for Dutch children who had suffered so much in the war. We had a meeting with a number of like-minded people from the embassy. One of them happened to have been a board member of the Christ Child Settlement House in Washington and therefore knew me and the work I had done there.

We decided to focus on the poorest section of The Hague. It was in the middle of the city, a warren of narrow alleys, bombed-out houses, and filth. According to the police, it was a haven for delinquents and black marketeers, a dangerous place where the police patrolled in pairs, if they went in at all. Most of the children and young people carried knives, which they had stolen from the retreating Germans. Stealing from Germans, and even killing them, had been considered heroic deeds during the war. Now that the war was over, some people continued to steal at every opportunity, mainly as a means of survival.

It was hard to know where to start, but we finally decided that the first thing we would try to do would be to open a playground for the children and youths in this neighborhood. These youngsters had been deprived of more than food, clothing, and shelter. They had been robbed of their childhood. We would try to give them some of it back.

It was decided that the others would concentrate on raising funds, while I would scout the neighborhood and try to get things started. I took my bicycle, filled my pockets with American chocolates, and ventured into the slum area. Right in the center of it, a bomb had destroyed about six little houses. Some of the walls were still standing, and the place was littered with glass and rubble. Once it was cleared, it would be just about the right size for what I had in mind.

The people living in the area were at first very suspicious of me. When I approached them with my plan and asked for their help, they thought that it was a ruse and that I was really after people dealing in black-market goods. But I came back every day, explaining, reassuring, and cajoling, and slowly I gained their trust. It may well have been the chocolates that did the trick; in any case, I finally got a group of boys together who agreed to pull down the ruined walls inside the bombed-out area. It took more chocolates to get them to stack the debris in large piles, which were then picked up by trucks loaned by the American Embassy. A bulldozer did the rest, and finally a steam-roller crushed the last of the stones and glass, pulverizing everything.

Our playground was ready, though *playground* is a rather grand word for the piece of dirty ground bordered on two sides by the walls of bombed-out buildings. One side was defined by a dilapidated fence, the fourth one was open to the street.

I had a volunteer working with me, a Red Cross nurse who had worked with children during the war. We wondered whether anyone would come. We need not have worried. As soon as the playground was officially declared open, it started to fill up with hordes of children of all sizes. They came—jostling each other, yelling, cursing, and fighting. They were dressed in rags, their torn clothes held together with rope and string. Some were barefoot. Some boys were wearing women's shoes, some girls had men's shoes on, but mostly they had only pieces of leather, cardboard, or even wood tied to their feet. We were amazed at their number. Where did they all spring from? How could that many children possibly live within these few blocks of damaged hovels?

At first the only equipment we had were some jump ropes and boxing gloves. These were an obvious attraction. I was immediately mobbed by children trying to get at them. They pulled at my arms and even jumped on my back, trying to grab the gloves. I still don't know how I kept my coat on or remained standing. My friend managed to lure the girls away by bringing out the jump ropes. I somehow got the boys into a rough circle before relinquishing the gloves to two of them. Before I could explain the rules, they went at each other. From the yelling and cheering of the spectators, I learned that these two boys were enemies. They had an old grudge to settle, relating to wartime thievery.

I quickly realized that they were fighting for real and that they would seriously hurt each other unless they were stopped. I also realized that they were in no mood to listen to any talk of sportsmanship. If I wanted to be heard, I needed to impress them in some way. But how to gain their attention and respect? There was only one way I could think of.

I got hold of the boys, and before they realized it, I had pulled the gloves off the hands of the smaller one and put them on myself. I really didn't know what to do next. The boy I faced was almost a foot taller than me and certainly much heavier. I told him that I would teach him to box properly, the way they did in America. I was grateful that I had watched some boxing matches on television with the youngsters at the Settlement House in Washington. I put up my hands and told him that the first thing one did was touch gloves. The group watching us had gone very quiet. I said a little prayer, and before he knew what was happening, I hit him hard on the chin. He went down. I took off my gloves and told him that it was not really fair for me to fight him, since I was obviously stronger and had more experience than he. He rubbed his chin and wanted to know how long I had had boxing lessons. "Not very long," I replied nonchalantly.

From that moment on, I had the boys' respect and my authority was established. Because we had no rope, I asked the boys to form a big square. I told them that I would match them for height and weight and that they would all get a turn at the gloves. But whoever broke the rules, such as hitting below the belt, would have to box with me. I kept each session very short, hoping that I could find a male volunteer to supervise them before I had to fight again. I was sure that I could not pull that particular trick off more than once!

Generous people gave us an American soccer ball. At that time, a soccer ball was an unheard-of luxury in Holland. Unfortunately, a ball did not have a very long life span, given the "shoes" our children wore and the condition of the ground. We soon needed a new one. This meant spending hours going from one office to another to justify our need. After weeks of knocking on office doors, we finally got official permission to purchase a ball—if we could find one. Then we had to scour the city until we actually located a ball, and then we were faced with the problem of how to pay for it. Somehow, we got the money.

The number of influential people eager to help us grew. The Australian ambassador provided us with swing sets for the younger children, as well as a seesaw. The American naval attaché brought over baseball equipment and spent time with the boys, teaching them the game. Embassies donated food so that we could provide the children with snacks. The playground became the social center of the whole neighborhood—and that brought problems with it.

We opened in the summer of 1946, and soon there was utter chaos. Not only children of all ages, but adolescents and even adults began to crowd the limited space. Robbed of a normal life by poverty and the war, the adults played like children, wanted to join in the soccer games, and went after the snacks we distributed. To keep a semblance of order we had to impose some kind of organization. We decided to open the playground at separate times for boys and girls until we could get more volunteers to help out with organized activities. Children under age seventeen were allowed to come during the day, older adolescents and adults in the evenings. We also extended our hours into the weekend.

The police had called me several times and warned me of the dangers to which I was exposing myself and the volunteers. The area we had chosen was a lawless and dangerous place, and the police foresaw all kinds of trouble. They were surprised, for example, that my bicycle had not yet been stolen, and thought that it would only be a matter of time until it disappeared. They asked me whether I realized that I was working with a bunch of gangsters. I had had no trouble, so far. What I saw were not gangsters, but desperately poor people who survived as best they could.

Nevertheless, I organized a meeting with everybody on the playground, children and adults, and told them that I knew about their criminal activities, their stealing, robbing, and black marketeering. I stressed that it was really none of my business but that anybody who wanted to continue being a member of the playground would have to stop stealing in this neighborhood. I promised that I would do my best to provide them with clothing and to help in any other way I possibly could, but I said that they would have to cooperate to that extent. They promised and, sure enough, the police reported that crime had suddenly decreased dramatically for miles around the area. I was sure that they still stole, simply going farther afield to do so, but as long as they kept to our agreement, I wasn't going to ask them about that.

Just about everybody was involved in some black-market activity or other, mostly dealing in stolen or forged food coupons. Every so often one would hear a whistle. This was a warning signal, indicating that the police were making a raid. One afternoon, police arrived on motorcycles, sirens screaming, and cordoned off the area. They started searching all of the houses.

A little three-year-old came running into the playground from one of the alleys and huddled against me. I took him into my arms, thinking that he had been frightened by this police invasion. When the police left, he gave me a big smile, put his hands in his pockets, and started pulling out fistfuls of stolen food and clothing coupons—the loot the police had obviously been after. Not only were his pockets full, some had even been shoved down the front of his dirty little shirt. When the warning whistle had sounded, his father had simply stuffed all his contraband into the child's clothes and sent him off to the playground. By that time I had become so much part of these people's lives that I felt like cheering his success in outsmarting the authorities.

One day when I was off duty, I was called and asked to come to the playground immediately, because there was trouble. I jumped on my bike and raced there as fast as I could go. When I got there, I found two of our male volunteers holding on to two of the bigger boys. They were perhaps seventeen and had gotten onto a fight, which ended with their pulling knives on each other. Luckily they had been interrupted before anyone was hurt. I asked them what had started such a serious fight. It turned out that one of them had been swinging on one of the swings meant for the little ones. When the other boy wanted a turn, he refused to get off.

My heart went out to them. These were children who had had to grow up too fast and had missed out on what should have been carefree and playful years. I asked them for their knives and they handed them over. I made another rule on the spot: nobody could come to the playground with any kind of weapon. Later, one of the embassies provided us with a set of larger swings, and soon everyone learned to take turns. The adults used the swings in the evenings and enjoyed them just as much as the teenagers.

It was clear to all of us that these people needed more than a place to play. We needed to expand our program, and for that we needed not only more money but also more trained volunteers who could work with this very special population, gain their trust, and help them in ways they could accept. We had raised enough money to be able to hire one full-time staff person. One of our most dedicated volunteers, a young woman who badly needed the money, was hired as director, and together we set up training programs for volunteers.

Fall had come, and with colder weather just around the corner, we became very concerned about the lack of warm clothing among our children. Underwear was unknown to our boys and girls. String took the place of buttons. What clothing they did have was generally ill fitting and so torn that it did not always cover them "decently," though nobody seemed to notice.

One little fellow came through the gate with nothing but a little cotton shirt on that was so short it didn't even cover his belly button. He was perhaps five years old. I called him over and told him to go home and put on some pants. One of the big boys heard me and said: "Aw, Miss Simons, you're not going to send him home for such a little thing, are you?" He told me that the boy's mother was in the hospital and that the oldest child, a ten-year-old girl, was taking care of the family. There were eight children in all, including a set of twins. In the meantime, the little boy had indeed gone home. He returned a short time later. He still had no pants on, but he had some newspaper wrapped around his lower body, tied with string. Nobody seemed to find this strange in the least, and of course he was allowed to stay.

With clothing in Holland rationed and almost unavailable, we racked our brains how to provide these people with the bare necessities to make it through the winter. Again, our American friends came to the rescue. They launched a clothing appeal among friends and relatives back in the States, and soon crates full of clothes started to arrive. Not all of them were exactly suitable for our purpose. We sorted out evening gowns and cocktail dresses, expensive suits, high-heeled shoes and fur coats and sold them to people who could afford such luxuries. They were much in demand, since even people who had not lost their money could not find clothes to buy. This clothing sale provided us with our main source of ready money.

Before distributing the rest, we decided to make home visits to ascertain people's needs. We were horrified to see the conditions under which these people lived. It was hard to believe that they could survive, let alone laugh and enjoy life. Sometimes there were ten, twelve, and even more people living in two or three tiny rooms with hardly any furniture.

I remember a visit with one of our poorest families. I happened to get there around noon. The staircase leading to their apartment was dark and narrow. Most of the steps were broken. The small room they lived in was so dark that at first I couldn't make out anything. All the windows had been broken during the bombings and were now covered with paper. The mother and one of the children were sick and lay in a corner of the room in the only bed. The oldest child, who could not have been more than ten, had done the cooking for their main meal of the day. It consisted of a mixture of sauerkraut and potatoes. There were no plates or utensils. Eight little heaps of food were put on the table, and the children ate them with their fingers. After they were done, they all stuck their hands in the pan and fought over the last shreds of food that stuck to it.

There was another family in whom I was particularly interested. In all, there were nine children between the ages of three and twenty-two. There was also a niece in her early twenties, who suffered from

TB. Whenever the weather permitted it, she was carried outside to sit in an easy chair in the alley. The mother had lupus, which had totally deformed one side of her face. I had only seen the father once, then he seemed to have disappeared. What struck me about this family was how well behaved these boys were. They were just about the only ones who never caused any trouble.

One day, I was invited to their home. The father had returned. It turned out that he had just been released from prison. I was offered tea. There was only one cup, and we took turns drinking from it. The father asked me how his sons had behaved in his absence. All six of them were lined up as if for inspection. I told him to ask the boys himself. They came to attention, almost like soldiers, and told their father that they had stayed out of trouble while he was away, and I was able to confirm this.

The father told me that he had been in and out of prison most of his life, mostly for stealing. This last time, he had gotten caught for dealing in the black market. With the money he had made, he had bought one of his sons a flower stand so he could make an honest living. With his next loot, he intended to provide a vegetable stand for another son. The only way he knew to provide for his children was by stealing and fencing things. He simply had to outsmart the police, which he mostly did. He was adamant that he would break the leg of any son who ever got caught stealing. He did not want them to follow in his footsteps and they better not try.

He dismissed his children and told me that there was something he wanted to show me. He carefully opened a large box and took a hat out of it. It was deep purple, with a heavy purple veil. He put the hat on his wife's head and gently pulled the veil over her face. He asked me if I knew why he had gotten this hat for her and then proceeded to answer his own question before I could think of anything to say. He said that he loved his wife, no matter what had happened to her face, but that they could not go out in public together without people staring at her and even averting their faces from her in disgust.

With this hat, he could take her out and she would not be humiliated. I wondered how it was possible to preserve a code of honor and to keep alive so much love and care in this dark overcrowded hole in the middle of a filthy slum.

Winter started early that year, and though we had some clothing, there was not enough for all the children. They came to the playground anyhow, most still in their thin rags, often without shoes or stockings. We were kept busy bandaging chilblains on heels and toes. Not only was the winter early, it also turned out to be one of the most severe in many years. I knew that we would need some kind of shelter to continue our work. What I had in mind was a kind of clubhouse.

We spent days in different offices to get the necessary permits to buy wood and nails. Everything was scarce, everything was rationed, and everywhere there was a pressing need for repairs and rebuilding. The officials we talked to couldn't believe their ears when they heard that we wanted these materials to build a shelter for a playground. After days of going from one official to another without much success, I got some of my friends at the American Embassy to intercede for us. The Dutch authorities knew only too well how much Holland owed to America, and a word in the right ear finally got us our permits.

What we ended up with was a room about twelve by twelve feet, built of cement and with two very small windows. It did not take much time to put it up, since we had many volunteers who helped pour the cement. When it was done it looked something like a bunker, but to us it was beautiful. We got pieces of old rugs to cover the floor, and one day, someone appeared with a little woodstove, which we fed with scraps of paper, twigs, and anything else that would burn.

Since there was only room for about twenty people at a time, we divided children and adults into small groups, who took turns at a variety of activities. I donated some of the knitting wool and needles I had brought with me from the States, and we also managed to scrounge around for needles and thread. The women knitted sweaters and learned to repair clothes. Even the boys started to learn knitting and other useful skills. Sometimes we cooked porridge or chocolate milk on our stove, delicacies they had not known for years. Someone got hold of a guitar, and we sang while our hands were busy.

I will never forget the first Christmas. The American naval attaché had gone to Belgium, where supplies were already more plentiful, and returned with sweaters, shoes, and toys. He and his wife had managed to get hold of an empty hall and had made arrangements for a Christmas dinner to be served there. It was impossible to get turkey, but there was plenty of other delicious food. For our people, it was like a dream. They ate and ate. Then we sang Christmas carols. Most of them had never been able to afford a proper Christmas celebration. They all returned home with warm sweaters and small parcels of food.

We struggled on through this hard winter and longed for spring and warmer weather. It eventually arrived, but I felt that what these children really needed was to be taken out of their unhealthy environment, at least for a while. I thought of ways we could make this happen. Then I remembered the camp we had organized for our children at the Christ Child Settlement House. Could we possibly pull something like this off for these children?

One of our benefactors owned a farm near the German border. I approached him with my plan, and he was willing to let us use it for a summer camp. I drove out and discussed logistics with the farmer. We were planning to have a group of boys and girls each spend two weeks in the country. He agreed that we could use the stables to sleep in, since the cattle would be outside during the summer.

As soon as the stables were empty, one of the volunteers and I went back to the farm to give them a thorough cleaning. We even whitewashed the walls. We put fresh straw in the loft where the youngsters would sleep. The stable itself would be both kitchen and dining room. We had neither tables nor chairs, but we carefully cleaned out the gutter that ran down the middle of the stable and propped a long plank over it, supported by four pieces of wood. Sitting on the floor, with their feet dangling into the gutter, the children would have a perfectly serviceable table.

We also wanted to do something for the mothers. Theirs was a life of unrelieved drudgery. They could not afford help to get away from their children for even a few hours, let alone take a brief vacation. And most of them had not had a proper childhood of their own. We decided to organize a day trip, with a picnic and a hayride. Volunteers were going to watch their younger children so they would get a proper break and not have to worry about their families. Baskets of food were provided by our staunch friend, the American naval attaché. We put hay and anything else that could cushion the ride in the back of a truck, and off we went, into the country. The women had a wonderful time, with lots of good food and games. I don't think any of them ever forgot this experience.

After our return from summer camp, we settled down for the fall program. I was approached by an organization devoted to child welfare that was interested in setting up similar playgrounds throughout the country, especially in neighborhoods with a high delinquency rate. It was to be a well-paying job, and my friends at the American Embassy with whom I had started our original project urged me to accept. I was tempted, but then I thought about the many well-trained social workers in Holland who had lived through the war here and were now in need of jobs. I didn't feel that it would be fair to take employment away from them.

I had begun to give some thought to my future. The playground project was well established and could continue without me. If I wanted to continue doing the kind of work I was interested in, I would have to get a social work degree. In all my past work, I had been guided mostly by common sense and by my lifelong ability to observe my environment and thus gain insight into people's needs. I had been lucky in finding jobs, usually before I went looking for them, and had generally been successful in everything I had undertaken. But I had also accepted any kind of job that was offered. With proper additional training, I would have more control over my life and the work I would be doing.

What I dreamed of was to get trained in America. For one thing, it was unlikely that a Dutch social work school would consider my application, since it was unusual to have students my age. For another, America was far advanced in the field of social work. But it would take a miracle to make this happen.

Sometimes in the early fall of 1947, I was at a cocktail party given by the American naval attaché. We discussed my work, and he asked me whether I was really serious about becoming a social worker. I told him that I certainly was and that, somehow, I would do it. He reached into his pocket and pulled out a ticket to the States. Handing it to me, he told me that he not only was prepared to pay for my trip but also was willing to finance my college costs. But I would have to make up my mind quickly. The reservation was for a week's time from now.

While I was still reeling from the shock, he got on the phone and called our mutual friend, the Dutch naval attaché in Washington. He told him that a friend wanted to talk to him and handed me the phone. Without further reflection, I told him that I was on my way back to America to study for a year or so. He was delighted and immediately invited me to stay with them as long as I wanted to.

A few days later I was on the plane to New York with absolutely no idea of how to get into college, but never doubting for a moment that, somehow, I would get my degree.

The two preceding chapters contain the very essence of Jeanne Simon's life: service where you are needed without regard to the cost to yourself; deep respect for human life in all of its manifestations; a tolerant and nonjudgmental attitude based on the understanding that, no matter what, people do the best they can, even though their behavior may be outside the norms acceptable to society; and deep empathy for parents overwhelmed by situations outside their control.

Also noteworthy is Jeanne's comment about how she dealt with emotions evoked by her return to a changed country. She describes the mutilated trees as "living things," "friends" who have been hurt. She can safely weep for them and for the loss of them, because they do not respond to her emotions. There is nothing unpredictable in this situation against which she has to guard.

Return to America, 1947
The social worker

There had been no question in my mind that I had to help my country after the war, and I had thrown myself into the relief work body and soul. But I didn't feel that I belonged there anymore. My family were strangers to me. They had gone on with their lives while I was away, and now they really didn't need me anymore. If I was to be honest, the decision to study in America was to some extent a way to separate myself from them without hurting their feelings. On the way to America, I experienced a sense of lightness and freedom. I was no longer bound by the expectations of others who had a claim on me.

The first thing I did after I returned to America was to get a list of colleges on the East Coast with good social work programs. There were about six or seven of them. Then I set out to visit each of them, to apply in person for admission. One after the other rejected me out of hand. Not only didn't I have proper university credentials, but the admissions officers were unfamiliar with the Dutch educational system and did not know how to evaluate the training I had received in Holland. Yet, with my teaching degree in early childhood education and the additional Montessori training, I had probably at least the equivalent of a bachelor's degree.

The last name on my list was Boston College. I went to talk to the dean there, telling her about my experiences and why I wanted to be a social worker. I also told her that Boston College was my last hope. She seemed interested in me. At least she didn't reject my application right away, as the others had done. After further discussion, she agreed to consider accepting me if I could find a professor within the department to supervise me. It was the semester break, but luckily one of the professors was working in her office. She interviewed me and agreed to be my sponsor. So in January of 1948, I became a graduate student in Boston.

I quickly felt comfortable in the program. I worked hard and was soon considered to be one of the top students in the department. I think one of the things that impressed the professors was my ability to quickly get past a case history and get to the person behind it. At first we only dealt with so-called paper cases. The professor would present a case based on a real or fictitious person's problems, and the students were encouraged to ask questions and offer suggestions on how one might approach such a case.

During the first such seminar I attended, the professor presented us with a case of a little boy who had accidentally choked his younger sister to death. What especially impressed the students was that despite her own grief, the mother had apparently been able to comfort and reassure her son. What struck me, however, were the relationships within the family, especially what sounded like an almost pathological closeness between mother and son. No one else picked up on that, so I finally ventured a timid question, not knowing whether I might be making a fool of myself. I said that I couldn't help wondering what would have happened if it had been the little girl who had accidentally killed her brother. I was convinced that in that case the mother could not have picked up her daughter and consoled her.

The class seemed surprised at this view of the case, and the professor looked at me so oddly that I was sure I had said something really dumb. She later told me that I had seen right through the case to its central element, but that this was only supposed to have been brought out much later in the class, through guided discussion.

During our second year we did field work. I was assigned to a mental health center, and I had some interesting challenges there. One of them was a woman who over the past years had been in and out of the center on a regular basis. Every staff member knew her and every student had been assigned to her. No one could do anything with her, yet time and again, she came back. She was a big, impressive-looking woman who always appeared to be angry and who therefore ended up being rejected by whoever was treating her. When she came in no one even greeted her anymore, and everyone shied away from working with her. Then, one day, it was my turn.

At our first meeting she sat there radiating hostility, and I knew right away that I wouldn't get to first base with her by using a traditional approach. Her anger did not bother me. I was sure that it was in part a reaction to the helplessness of the people who had tried to work with her before. That she always came back was a clear enough indication that there was something she needed to deal with. At first I didn't question her in any way but just tried to be as friendly as possible and just engaged in casual conversation with her. As we chatted, she mentioned her child who came to the center and the finger painting he had done with his therapist.

I knew then and there that I had found my opening. I told her I thought she would be very good at that herself and invited her to bring an apron with her next time she came to see me, so we could do some painting. She did come in with an apron and, as promised, we painted. Her paintings were an outpouring of extreme anger. Naturally, I did not comment on that. I just accepted it. The painting session seemed to have broken the ice.

After that she started to open up, and only a few visits later she told me about the hatred she felt toward her husband. He had TB when they met but had not told her. He also squandered their money. She felt terribly betrayed by him and didn't want to have children with him. Every time she got pregnant, she had an abortion. Finally, she decided to carry one baby to term, not because she had changed her mind but because she wanted to make sure that even after she was dead there would be someone left to hate her husband.

I commented that she must have cared for this man an awful lot, because you could only hate that much if you had loved very deeply.

At this, she broke down and started to cry and talk as if a dam had burst. I saw her one more time, but I felt that she needed to be in more highly trained hands, so I transferred her to a very sensitive woman psychiatrist with whom she reportedly made good progress.

Another case I remember vividly involved the parents of a child being treated at the center. They were well-to-do, articulate people who sat in my office side by side, very properly and attentively, smiling politely and answering every question I asked. But despite their outward helpfulness, I got the strong feeling that they were present in body only. Where they were sitting was a sort of empty space. In an attempt to understand them better, I asked permission from my supervisor to make a home visit. It was granted, and my clients invited me for dinner.

They had a very nice, well-kept home. The food was good and it was presented nicely. Yet the whole time I was there, I felt extremely uncomfortable. At first I couldn't put my finger on what was bothering me. Then I realized that what was missing were emotions. There was talk but no real communication, no three-way conversation. The couple was very polite to each other, they did everything correctly, but even when they smiled at each other, nothing flowed between them. There was absolutely no feeling. I told my supervisor that these people had no emotions, neither positive nor negative ones, that there was no give-and-take between them, that each member of the family, including the child, seemed separated from the other by a cold space within each of them.

I was surprisingly shaken by this experience. It wasn't until much later that I realized that I had encountered my first autistic adults. I know now that I must have recognized something of myself in them, without knowing what it was. I saw too much. I knew without knowing. Yet at the time I knew nothing about autism—very few people did—and I did not realize until many years later that I myself was different from others in some very significant ways, one of which was my difficulty with emotions. I had learned to deal with this difficulty as I had learned to walk and talk, and it never occurred to me to wonder how other people handled the problems attached to relationships.

As I was very much aware of my obligations to my benefactor, I finished my course work in record time and graduated after a year and a half, in June of 1949, with a master's degree in social work. Through the work I had done at the Christ Child Settlement House, I had connections to a psychiatrist in Washington. In fact, he had written one of the required letters of recommendation for me when I applied to social work schools. When he heard that I was about to graduate, he wrote and offered me a job at an institution he was connected with.

The place, called Children's House, was a privately owned outpatient treatment facility for emotionally and behaviorally disturbed children in Washington, DC. It was run by a mother-daughter team and, at the time I joined the staff, was already financially very unstable. Shortly afterward it was on the point of bankruptcy, and the owners wanted to close it down.

Genevieve, one of the other social workers on the staff, and I believed there was a great need for a place like Children's House and offered to take over running it. Since we could not afford to pay any salaries, the rest of the staff had to leave. This included support staff as well as professional staff, so we ended up doing everything ourselves. My friend Genevieve was a good businesswoman and did all the administrative work. I worked with the children. The other tasks, we split between us. Genevieve was independently wealthy and did not need to worry about getting paid, and she invited me to live with her until we started making enough of a profit so I could get a salary again.

The center had a good reputation, referrals kept coming in, and with better management our financial situation slowly began to improve, so that after a while we were ready to expand and to move to a larger place. There we continued to do well, and eventually we moved again, this time to a complex on Nebraska Avenue that had been especially designed and built for us. One building housed the outpatient services, one a social agency we worked with, and a third a residential program we had newly added. Originally children had only been seen individually. There had been a brief attempt at offering a day program, but it had folded because it had been too expensive for most parents.

This is a pivotal chapter in both Jeanne's journey toward her pioneering work and her self-discovery. It also, once again, shows her dogged persistence in getting to a goal she has set herself.

In all of Jeanne's previous work with individual children and groups of children, her approach—as we have seen—was guided by her training as a Montessori teacher and her own philosophy of working with the strength of children in her care and letting them lead the way. Her clinical training at Boston College expanded her knowledge, but it mainly seems to have allowed her to apply her uncanny ability to cut to the root of a problem in ever more severe cases.

But it was also at Boston College that she had a first premonition of her own autism. She states quite clearly that her wish to study in America was in good part fueled by her need to distance herself from her family, who, during her enforced absence during World War II, "had become strangers." She states that getting training abroad was "a way to separate myself from them without hurting their feelings." But hitherto, she had never questioned why she had such difficulties with emotions, saying that she had learned to deal with it "as I had learned to walk and talk."

When she encountered the parents of a patient who seemed to be missing emotions in their interactions with their child and between themselves, the experience deeply shook her, and in retrospect she thought she must have recognized something of herself in these people without, at the time, knowing what it was or indeed knowing anything about autism. Her ignorance of autism while recognizing something that resonated within her persisted into the early years she worked with children with autism at Children's House in Washington and later at Linwood, as she describes in the next chapter.

Lee, Martin, and the miracle worker

Lee was the first youngster officially diagnosed with autism that Jeanne Simons worked with in an inpatient setting—albeit that of her own home. Martin was one of a group of children at Children's House with such severe problems that they seemed headed for a life in an institution. Some of them are described in *The Hidden Child*. Lee and Martin stand out, not only because of the severity and seeming hopelessness of their cases, but also because the treatment Jeanne devised for them exemplifies both her treatment philosophy and the methods that led to the successes at Linwood.

Lee

I started out doing individual therapy at Children's House, then I revived a modified day program for acting-out youngsters, which I ran year-round. One day in the summer of 1950, a couple brought in their eleven-year-old son for an interview. When the boy was three, Dr. Leo Kanner had diagnosed him as autistic. He lived in a private residential institution for emotionally disturbed youngsters. His parents took him home as often as possible, but the older he got, the more unmanageable he became. He was extremely self-destructive, with scars all over his face and hands from his own scratching. They were hoping that I could help them with him while he was home for a one-month vacation.

While I was talking with his parents, I observed Lee. He seemed unaware of his surroundings or of me. He kept moving around the room, flipping a key chain from one hand to the other. His mother talked about his temper tantrums, his compulsions, and how difficult he was. I looked at him and said: "Lee, we are talking about you. Your mother would like me to try to help you." Lee did not give any indication that he was hearing me. His mother said that he could not understand what I was saying to him and that he had no awareness of other people. Nevertheless, as we continued the conversation, I reminded Lee from time to time that we were talking about him.

As Lee and his parents prepared to leave, I looked again at his scratched and scarred face and arms. My heart went out to this deeply troubled, helpless child and his desperate parents. I promised to see him as often as possible. They left, but Lee became upset as soon as he went out the door. His mother brought him back again. He didn't look at me but just stood there, scratching his face and looking very upset. I put my hand on his head and said: "Try to show me what upsets you." Lee kissed me and mumbled: "I want you to be my mother." I replied: "I will try to be a good friend to you, Lee." He smiled and walked out without another look.

During the following month, I saw Lee whenever possible, afternoons and weekends. Sometimes his parents called me late at night because he was so upset. Somehow I was able to reach him and quiet him down a little, although I never understood what he was upset about. As the month went on, I found that I understood some of what Lee was saying in his garbled way. I also found that I could set limits on some of his most severe compulsions and reduce the frequency and intensity of his temper tantrums.

Finally, Lee's vacation ended, and his family was preparing to send him back to his institution. The day before he was to leave, he came up to me and told me in his awkward way that he wanted to live with me. I will never know what came over me. After talking to Lee's parents, I rented a big farmhouse with lots of land around it and moved into it with Lee and with a young couple, a medical student and his wife, who were to help both with the farm and with Lee. I also managed to get Lee into one of the small groups at Children's House.

As soon as I had set everything up, I panicked. I knew next to nothing about children like Lee and had no way of knowing what I had gotten myself into. I went to talk to Dr. Kanner at the Johns Hopkins School of Medicine, the psychiatrist who had been the first to identify autism as a separate syndrome and who had known Lee since he was three years old. I hoped that he would give me his blessing for the task I was about to undertake. When I told him what I had done, he looked at me in disbelief. He thought for a moment, puffing on his huge cigar, and finally he spoke. "It's worth a try," he said. I felt as if a great weight had been lifted from me. I'll never forget the support and advice Dr. Kanner gave me during the incredible year that followed.

Shortly afterward, Lee moved in with me. Almost immediately, I got a taste of what was to come. Lee found an old cowbell and ran through the house ringing his "freedom bell"—freedom from the institution he had been in, freedom from people he was afraid of. I showed him his room, which opened into my own. When he saw it, all the happiness left his face. He stared at the door leading to the room, then he clawed at his face, bit his hands, screamed, and hit the door with his head. I asked him what was wrong but he didn't seem to hear me. He just scratched, clawed, bit, and hit himself even harder.

I looked at the door to see what might be wrong: The color? The knob? It was just an ordinary door. Then I noticed the keyhole. Was Lee perhaps afraid of being locked up? I told him that there was no key, that I could not lock his door. His attacks on himself became still more violent. He stared at the keyhole. I was right, he was afraid of being locked in. I racked my brain for a way to assure Lee that I could not lock him up, and finally came up with a solution. That afternoon, we sawed the door in half, so that it worked like a Dutch door. This gave us both an illusion of privacy, but it assured Lee that the door could not be locked. Years later, Lee told me that this incident was crucial in gaining his trust.

When it was time to go to bed, Lee insisted on taking about twenty different objects to bed with him. One of them was the key chain that he never parted from. The others included a worn-out teddy bear and several small beads. The next morning, it was difficult to get Lee going. He had an elaborate series of rituals he had to go through to get dressed. The second night, Lee looked in his room and immediately fell apart. He screamed, banged his head, and gagged. I realized that one of his objects must be missing. Crawling on the floor, I looked everywhere—under the bed, behind the radiator—and when at last I found the little lost bead, I was exhausted.

I also realized that Lee could make me even more compulsive than he was. I knew that I would rather search for hours to find what he had lost than to live through his screaming and self-aggression. So the next morning, after Lee got up, I took all his objects and arranged them neatly on his dresser. Before he went to bed that night, I told him that those were not my objects, so *he* was responsible for them. For a few mornings I helped him line them up on the dresser so they would not get lost. After a while he no longer lost his objects, and I was gradually able to help him reduce the number of objects he took to bed.

From the first day Lee lived with me, he demanded every minute of my time. He endlessly babbled about whatever was on his mind, asked me for help, and flew into a rage when I could not give him immediate attention, or if the telephone rang and I had to answer it. I knew that I would be drained of all mental and physical energy within a week if I allowed things to continue this way. I also knew that if Lee was ever to be able to adjust to life at home, he would have to be able to occupy himself and live in a more normal environment. I set up one room in the house where Lee could discuss his problems and where I would be his therapist. While we were in that room, he had my full attention, and no interruptions were allowed. However, at other times, and in the rest of the house, I was Lee's friend, not his therapist. Lee accepted this. He called me "Miss Simons" during the therapy sessions, but between sessions, he called me by my first name.

One of Lee's compulsions had to do with birthdays. He insisted on knowing everyone's birthday. He even stopped strangers in the street and demanded to know the date they were born. He became very upset and self-aggressive if people did not answer him. Lee had a built-in calendar in his head, and he could tell what day of the week a person had been born on if they told him their age and birth date. He was never wrong. He never revealed his own birthday, however, and if someone asked about it, he would often fall to the floor, roll his head from side to side, and gag. His fascination with dates was so extreme that he would pick newspapers out of the trash can, or even out of an open fire, just to read the date on them.

It was several months before I got a clue to this fixation on birthdays and dates. Lee had started to tell me stories that he wanted me to type for him. He talked in a monotone, very rapidly, never stopping between words. When he dictated to me, he spelled out the words instead of saying them. He spelled faster than I could type, and he never made a spelling mistake. I had to ask him to slow down so that I could follow him, and he did. Later, he decided on his own to start pronouncing the words instead of spelling them, running the words together so that every sentence was one long word.

All of Lee's stories concerned events in his early childhood. They contained the most minute details of people's clothing, the number of knocks on a door, replays of conversations, names, etcetera. I asked him to put dates to the memories, which he was easily able to do. Then I noticed that the stories he dictated took place at earlier and earlier dates. If the dates were correct, he was remembering things from a time when he was two years old or younger. Sometimes he would refuse to give me a date, saying that it was too long ago. The dates he did give me had him remembering things ever further back. I was puzzled. I had never known Lee to be wrong about dates, yet the dates he gave me took us back to a time before he was a year old. If I asked him if he was sure about a date, he would wring his hands, roll his head back and forth violently, gag, and scratch his forehead open with his fingernails.

One day Lee dictated a story that consisted mostly of babbling and a few baby words, along with sounds of doors closing, a train going by, and the words adults use when they address a baby. While telling the story, Lee gagged and his breathing became labored. I was afraid that he might be about to have an asthma attack or a seizure. I told him to stop dictating and save the story till later, but he refused. As he continued telling the story, he became more and more agitated. Finally, he mumbled a date when these events were supposed to have taken place. It was before he was born. I knew that I had a mystery to solve.

I immediately set up an appointment with Lee's father. I asked him about Lee's birthday. He seemed perturbed and wanted to know why I was interested in his son's birthday. I told him that I felt that Lee's compulsions about dates might have something to do with his own birthday. "Miss Simons," he said, "No one knows about this except Lee's mother, his grandmother, and me." He told me that when Lee was about three years old, the family moved to a neighborhood where no one knew them. Because Lee was so tiny, they told everyone that he was only eighteen months old, so people would not ask what was wrong with him. This meant that Lee was really thirteen rather than eleven.

The next day I told Lee about his real birthday. He did not show much of a reaction, only wondering whether he had "lost" two years. But he seemed relieved and almost immediately lost his intense compulsion about dates and birthdays. He still asked people about their birthdays but did not insist on an answer. For the first time he also enjoyed his own birthday when it came around. I figured out that Lee's obsession with dates must have arisen from the fact that his was the only birthday in the world that did not fit his built-in calendar. His parents had told him what day of the week he was born on, but it didn't square with his calculations for the year he was given. When he found out that he was really two years older, the date finally fit.

Lee had many other compulsions, too. He would announce, for example, that he was going to play a record a set number of times. The number was always in the hundreds. He would play the first few grooves over and over again until he got to the number he had specified. I began to count to see if this was true and found that he was always accurate. If something interrupted him before he finished the number he had specified, he got very upset.

Lee also had a set of rituals around getting up in the morning. He had to run around, pace up and down, move his chair, and do a series of complex actions to get going. These rituals took about an hour every morning, but he usually performed them cheerfully and was then ready for the day. One day, however, Lee woke up and seemed very upset. He refused to talk, banged his head, and wrung his hands. He took much longer than usual to get dressed and stayed upset for most of the day. I had no idea what had gotten him into such a state.

About a month later, he again woke up looking anxious and banging his head. This time I decided he needed help. I picked him up, put him on a chair, and dressed him. I expected a tantrum; here I was, breaking in on his cherished rituals. Instead, he gave a big sigh and mumbled: "You should have done this fifteen minutes ago, and you should have done it on November 12" (which was the day he had awakened in an anxious mood the first time). Years later, Lee explained to me that his rituals were designed to help him get away from his dreams—good or bad. On the two occasions where he had been so agitated, he had not been sure whether his dream had been good or bad, and he needed my help to get away from these dreams.

As time went on Lee's compulsions gradually diminished, and we developed a good relationship, although he never established eye contact with me—or with anybody else, for that matter. He also didn't want to be touched. For many months I did not allow friends to visit me on the farm, feeling that I wanted to give Lee the chance to be the only child and to assure him of my undivided attention. I did go out, occasionally, to see friends, leaving Lee with the young couple who shared the house, and Lee accepted this. However, I finally decided it was time to have friends come to visit us. I invited a couple I knew to spend the weekend with us.

I told Lee about the upcoming visit and he asked me all kinds of questions: Would they like him? Would I go out with them and leave him? I assured him that this was his house, too, and that we would include him in anything we did. He seemed relieved and seemed to look forward to the visit.

The day before my friends came, I was preparing a pudding when Lee came into the kitchen and lay down on the floor. He was very pale. He gagged and rolled his eyes back. It looked as if he was going to have one of his seizures. "Miss Simons," he said, "I am very sick. I am going to die." He looked as if he might be serious, but I said: "Lee, please don't die on the kitchen floor. Why don't you stretch out on the living room couch? I'll be with you in a minute. Don't go upstairs, you are definitely too sick to climb stairs." Lee sat straight up. His color came back, and I could see that he was out of danger.

When I came into the living room, he was on the couch, playing a record. I sat down quietly next to him. Ten minutes later he asked me: "What was that awful feeling I had?"

"Maybe you are jealous," I replied.

"Is jealous a feeling I get when you make pudding for your friends?" He did not wait for an answer. When my friends came and Lee saw that he was still accepted as part of the family, he lost his anxiety and learned to welcome further visitors.

During the year at the farm Lee's seizures greatly diminished. He had a theory of why this might have happened. One day, when we were working through one of his many compulsions, he told me that now this was "off his mind." He explained to me that things he worried about used to go from his mind down to his stomach, where they gave him seizures. Since I had been working with him, he said, many of the things he had been anxious about were finally off his mind and no longer caused trouble. He speculated that they might have "gone out the window." Along with his seizures, Lee's asthma tantrums almost totally disappeared, and he was no longer self-aggressive.

Lee returned home after a year at the farmhouse, and I moved back into an apartment. Lee initially had severe problems adjusting to his family, and I saw him once a week or more for several months. After that, he learned to get along with his family and lived at home rather comfortably until he was twenty-one. His parents were even able to take him on a trip to Europe. When he was twenty-one, Lee moved to a village for the handicapped, where he adapted very well. He baked bread there and was very proud of it. He came to visit me when he was home for holidays, and he was always glad to see me. Lee died of a brain hemorrhage when he was twenty-six, still looking much younger than his age.

LIVING WITH LEE had taught me a great deal. I was especially impressed by how completely children with problems as severe as his could take over the family. They demand total attention, need constant supervision, and disrupt all normal activities and relationships. On the other hand, my work with Lee had also convinced me that with a great deal of patience they could be reached and that even their most bizarre behavior seemed to serve a purpose and was not simply something to be either suppressed or catered to. I began to think that there were many children who had been given up on and eventually shut away in institutions who might be helped with the right kind of intensive treatment. Most of them were never even considered for an outpatient program. At Children's House, too, there were guidelines for children accepted for treatment. The very young disturbed ones, especially if they also appeared retarded, were not even seen for evaluation but were referred to Rosewood, a state hospital.

I saw the desperation of the parents who could not find a program for their children and had to institutionalize them for lack of other options, and I remembered Lee and his distress at the thought of having to go back to the institution where he had not been helped. Once the Children's House had moved to its new quarters on Nebraska Avenue, I proposed that I be allowed to put together a group of these children and try to work with them. At first I had only three or four children between the ages of three and seven, but there was obviously a great need for this type of program, so before long we had sixteen children. As the group grew in size, I had one assistant, and later a teacher came in for an hour to help out.

I did not know anybody who worked with children who were this young and as severely disturbed. Not knowing what to expect, I had no particular program in mind, but I had stocked the room with toys I thought might interest them. The first day the children were brought in they didn't even give these toys a glance. They did not look at me, either, acknowledge my presence in any way, or take any notice of each other. Each one seemed preoccupied with their own concerns and activities, turned inward and separated from the others by some invisible space that enclosed them and protected them from intrusions by the outside world.

I walked around the room, gently touching each child. They shrank away. I sat on the floor among them, watching them, and racked my brain, thinking of all the books I had read about disturbed, psychotic, and brain-damaged children. Apparently somebody had forgotten to write about *these* children. I realized only many years later that somebody actually had written about them. But even though I knew Dr. Kanner through my work with Lee, it took many years of working with these children before I made the connection between the behaviors I observed in them and those presented by Lee and the other, older, youngsters like him. Dr. Kanner had studied a group of such children whose condition he had given the name *early infantile autism* only six years earlier.

Most of the children immediately set up some sort of boundary for themselves beyond which they rarely moved. Some of them appeared passive, sitting perfectly still and staring into space for long periods. At such times they did not react when their names were called or they were talked to. It was as if they were deaf. Others seemed wrapped up in repetitive activities, as if in an invisible cloak. They would cling to the compulsions with quiet stubbornness and at times with a sense of desperation, almost as if their lives depended on it. They would get anxious, to the point of panic, if their compulsions were interfered with.

Physical closeness was clearly uncomfortable for these children. Some actively avoided it, some tolerated it but appeared stiff and unyielding as if made of wood, and some ignored it, either not seeming to notice the closeness of another person or swatting at a touching hand as one swats at an annoying fly.

Their need for being safely isolated in a space of their own was so great that some of them seemed to want to physically disappear. They tended to hide in any available space—in closets and under tables—and if nothing else was at hand, they would turn a box upside down and fold themselves away under it. People who came to observe our group were often faced with nothing but the sight of one or two boxes moving around the room.

The children had come with a variety of labels: brain damaged, retarded, schizophrenic. That was no help at all when it came to dealing with them. But even if we had had the correct diagnosis, it would not have made any difference to our work with them. Each of these children was unique, with a distinct personality and own way of struggling with life. Each of them presented a new, fascinating challenge.

I wrote about many of these children in *The Hidden Child*. Here I want to tell about the one I called our "littlest angel." I tell Martin's story because he stayed with us for most of my time at Children's House and also because his story both makes it easier to understand why it was thought that this type of child could not be reached and shows the time and patience it takes to help such a child move even the smallest step forward.

Martin

Martin came to Children's House in October 1951, when he was not yet five years old. He was tiny, barely over three feet tall, and he weighed only about twenty-seven pounds. His birth had apparently been normal but he immediately had a severe feeding problem. He would have starved to death if his mother had not spent hours and hours around the clock giving him his bottle. He refused to be fed by his father and only accepted one particular nipple. When that finally gave out, he refused the bottle altogether and had to be introduced to baby food. This was extremely difficult, since Martin refused any kind of variety and for months and months would only eat one kind of food.

Except for feeding, Martin was an easy baby. He made no demands whatsoever, he did not cry, he did not ask for attention, he seemed perfectly satisfied to be left in his crib or playpen for hours on end. In fact, he seemed totally unaware of people. He did not respond when his parents talked to him, never looked at them, never smiled or imitated anyone. The only thing that seemed to interest him was any kind of small object with a screw top. He would sit by himself for hours, unscrewing the top and screwing it on again, unwilling to give up the object he was playing with.

Martin was a year and a half old when the pediatrician told his parents to consult a psychiatrist. The doctor was concerned because the child responded so differently from other babies he saw in his practice. Martin did not seem aware of the doctor or the instruments and did not even show any reaction when he was given a shot. It was as if he didn't feel the pain. At the age of two Martin was officially diagnosed with primary infantile autism. Outpatient therapy was started on a once-a-week basis, which was later increased to three times a week. At first Martin seemed to be making some progress, but then he suddenly regressed. The parents were advised to suspend further treatment until he was older.

By now, the parents' anxiety was fully aroused. They went from one place to another looking for help, but without success. Then they heard that an attempt was being made at Children's House to work with children like Martin, and they brought him to us, hoping against hope that we would be able to do something for him.

When I first saw Martin, he reminded me of a deer. He had a delicately formed, graceful body and big brown eyes, which seemed to look inward. The expression on his almost transparent face never changed. It seemed to be a mixture of sadness, great wisdom, and fear. His mother brought him into the room holding him by the hand. I took his hand from her and she left. There was no indication that he had noticed. He seemed to be in a dream. I took off his jacket and he quickly settled down in the middle of the room and started to play with the small screw-top bottle he had brought with him. He was totally focused on it and did not seem to see anything or anybody else.

The space he occupied seemed defined by invisible borders beyond which he rarely ventured. Once in a while he would put the bottle down and walk in a circle around it, moving his arms and hands in a most graceful way and making what sounded like expressions of pleasure, though the sad expression on his face never changed. If his bottle top accidentally rolled beyond the boundaries of his imaginary circle, he would reach for the nearest adult hand and, holding on to it, would get it back. He would only let go of the hand once he was safely back in his space. These were the only occasions when Martin's expression changed, taking on an intense anxiety that disappeared as soon as he had his top back.

As the weeks went by Martin slowly expanded his original boundaries, until they encompassed the whole room. He did this by holding on to someone's hand and carefully pacing off ever-larger circles within which he could move freely. If he had to move beyond this space, for example to go to the bathroom or to go home, he became agitated, and he could only do it by clinging to someone's hand. After he had conquered most of the room, I thought that he was ready to be introduced to outside play. I carried him into the yard. At first he clung to me, and then he immediately set up a safe space, which he expanded the way he had done indoors. As he freed himself from his confining boundaries, he also became less obsessed with bottles and became interested in other objects.

Like many of our children, Martin liked to hide in small places. Whenever there was a box big enough for him to hide under, he would take it into his space and crawl under it. As he expanded his area, he would carry the box with him. To test his reaction, I would sometimes put my foot into his box. He would simply remove it, as if it was an unwanted object.

After about three months with us, Martin went through a strange ritual that somehow reminded me of a reenactment of the birth process. Shortly after this, I again put my foot into his box. He removed it as usual, then hesitated, moved the box out of my reach, and came up to me, making it clear that he wanted to be picked up. When I complied, he looked straight at me for the first time ever, and then, quick as a flash, he scratched me furiously. He had clearly made the connection between me and the foot that was in his way.

After that when he needed help, he was no longer satisfied with *any* hand—he definitely looked for *my* hand. It was the first indication that he seemed not only to realize the difference between inanimate objects and body parts but also to recognize that they belonged to different people, with a definite preference for one person. He had taken the first step toward developing an ability to relate to people.

When he wanted something, Martin would take my hand, guide it toward the desired object, and, using my hand like a tool, have me get it for him. It took a whole year before he could take what he wanted by himself, and several months more before he dared take anything without needing to be reassured that it was all right for him to have it.

Once Martin had established a first relationship with me, he started looking directly at me whenever he wanted something. He began to insist on a lot of cuddling, and when I held him, he made all the sounds one hears from very small babies. His face became more expressive and he looked relaxed and satisfied when being cuddled. From an evasive sprite, Martin became the cuddliest little child, but as he became more alive he also began to show signs of anger when something displeased him. He expressed his anger by scratching me, which he did both when I did not immediately understand what he wanted and when others bothered him—for example, when another child interfered with his play.

When he had first started taking notice of others, he had reacted to their intrusions by wringing his hands, turning in circles, and shaking his head furiously or banging it against a hard surface. But more and more often he would fling himself at me and cover me with scratches, as if holding me responsible for the harm done to him. It was impossible to avoid him. He was fast as lightning and launched himself at me like a little tiger. My hands suffered the most. One day I simply couldn't take any more and put gloves on. Before I knew what was happening, Martin had lifted the leg of my blue jeans and inflicted deep scratches on my leg.

Increasingly Martin's activities were aimed at getting attention not just from me, but from everyone around him. One way he managed to do this was by throwing objects. At first he did this only when he was upset about something, but more and more he seemed to do it for the pure pleasure of it, and it became a daily activity. Since the objects he threw were generally small ones, we tried not to interfere too much with his pleasure. But Martin seemed to be determined to get us to react.

The objects he chose became larger and larger. He had a really naughty sparkle in his eyes as he checked whether we were watching before he threw one of them. Once, when he was threatening to throw a big truck, he laughed out loud as two staff members converged on him to prevent it. It was so wonderful to see and hear him laugh and to see his big eyes alive with that devilish sparkle that we really didn't want to stop or restrict him. But his activities were becoming dangerous to the other children, so we tried to divert him before he grabbed for something to throw. Anybody who saw Martin poised would interrupt anything they were doing to distract him. It quickly became clear that we could not continue to give him this disproportionate amount of attention. The time had come to set some limits on his behavior.

We had a little playhouse in the room, which Martin often used as a retreat. One morning, his entry into the room was preceded by his lunchbox, which popped open, with shards from his baby food jars flying all over the room. He watched staff members scurry to clean up the mess before one of the other children could hurt themselves, and every so often he burst out in peals of laughter. I told him that it was too early in the day to start throwing things, and that he would have to spend some time sitting in the playhouse if he didn't quiet down a little. He looked at me as if he understood and agreed with me, but another crash in the playroom and a burst of laughter told me that I was wrong.

I took Martin by the seat of his pants and sat him down in the cabin. At first he looked at me in a puzzled way, then he tried to charm me with a smile. I explained to him again why he was being "punished." He sat down on the little bench and started to cry. These were the first tears we had ever seen him shed. He made no attempt to leave the cabin, and there were no signs of anger or anxiety. It almost seemed as if he had been waiting for someone to set some limits on his behavior. The throwing episodes diminished, but he continued to test the limits. He seemed to have an inexhaustible store of ways to keep us busy.

Over time his need for attention seemed to decrease, and he also started to form relationships with staff members other than myself. It was only when he was in great distress or trying something out for the first time that he insisted on being with me.

In more than two years with us, Martin had made enormous progress. He had gone through several phases of first accepting, then rejecting, and again accepting new foods, and by now he had a more varied diet, though he still only ate things in pureed form. By dipping my finger into milk and putting a few drops on his lips, I had also gotten him to drink milk. He still would not play with others, but now if someone interfered with his activities he came for help instead of becoming upset and hurting himself or me, as he had done previously. He had also expanded his activities, including a phase of water play. But then he suddenly became very compulsive again and returned to his preoccupation with screw-top objects.

He seemed tense and anxious. For days in succession he would cry or throw himself against a hard surface. One moment he wanted to be cuddled, the next he would kick and scratch. I had noticed that his progress was uneven and that periods of regression usually preceded some major step forward. So, when it happened this time, I watched him carefully to see what changes he might be ready for.

I noticed some new behaviors around food. He would take sandwiches, smell them, then throw them away. He would choose his baby food and, as soon as he had it, smash the jar. I had the feeling that he was ready to eat solid foods. I took a tiny amount of some food and forced it into his mouth. He resisted, but instead of his customary scratching or kicking, he chewed and swallowed it. Every day he would come and indicate that he wanted food, and although he showed some resistance, he always ate it in the end. Eventually he started to eat solids by himself and after a second summer spent with us in a residential summer camp, he stopped having a feeding problem and ate normal meals with fork and spoon, sitting at the table with the other children.

It was also during that summer that he took a baby bottle, filled it with milk and very solemnly drank part of it through the nipple. Then he emptied the rest of the milk into a cup, handed me the bottle and drank the rest of the milk from the cup. This was the first time Martin had drunk from a nipple since he had refused the bottle when he was four months old, and the episode came after several weeks of doll play in summer camp.

His mother had dropped him off with two stuffed animals without whom he refused to go to sleep. The first evening we had put the animals on his bed, but that night Martin "drowned" them in the bathtub and then buried them deep in the trash can. The next night he took a doll to bed with him, and he also carried it around with him during the day, tenderly bathing it, putting it to bed, and feeding it water from a doll's nursing bottle. His play activities expanded further, and after a while he began noticing the live animals we had, watching them for hours and petting and feeding them.

Six months later he became very compulsive again, gave up most of his play activities, and seemed to regress once more. This time I had no idea what, if any, kind of gain he would make. He seemed desperately anxious, and my arms were often bleeding from his scratches. This period lasted for about two weeks; then, one morning when he came in, he rushed up to the other children, hugged them, gave them toys, and tried to sit on the same chair with them. Wherever he went, he tried to drag another child after him like a rag doll. As always, after he had gone through a period of regression, he appeared to be a changed child. This time, his leap forward had propelled him into making genuine contact with others and to take pleasure in interacting with them.

Once he had made this breakthrough, he was also able to start sharing me with the other children. He would still stop what he was doing and come to me for a reassuring hug when he saw another child climb on my lap, but he would not get upset and would quickly return to his play. Later, he would even take a child who was upset or crying by the hand and bring him to me, pushing him on my lap. He took one child who had thrown himself on the floor in a temper tantrum into an adjoining room and "read" a book to him. He made all sorts of sounds, moved his head from one side to the other as if following the printed text with his eyes, and turned pages at regular intervals. Once in a while he would peek over the book at the other youngster, wipe his nose off with a Kleenex tissue, and then continue "reading" until the child calmed down.

The first words he spoke also came after a period of heightened anxiety and seeming distress. He started repeating words, but for several months he could only do it through a piece of paper he rolled up or another object with a hole in it, which he held it in front of his mouth and spoke through.

MARTIN'S BEHAVIOR AND PROGRESS in many ways exemplify what we saw in this special group of youngsters. What impressed me was that while change came very slowly, it was nevertheless possible. Children who had been dismissed as hopeless and who might have been consigned to lifelong residential care showed signs of growth, demonstrated an ability to relate, and started to communicate. But regardless of their progress, they continued to be so difficult to deal with that their parents were often incapable of keeping them at home while at the same time holding a job or leading any kind of normal family life.

The need for a specialized residential treatment facility became more and more apparent to me. Also, Children's House had changed its policy, deciding to put its resources into diagnostically more hopeful groups of children. So, I had to make a choice. I would either have to give up working with these children or strike out on my own.

Linwood, 1955 I2

I knew that I could not abandon these children, and I also felt a strong obligation to their desperate parents. They promised to help in any way they could to enable me to continue the work with their children. Friends and professionals I was working with at Children's House also offered encouragement, so in 1955 I decided to look around for a place where I could open a small residential program.

The property I had in mind had to meet a number of criteria. It had to be reasonably close to Washington, where most of our children lived. It had to be large enough to provide plenty of room inside and out. It had to be somewhat secluded, without close neighbors who might be disturbed by a group of unruly and often noisy youngsters, and it had to be secure, to assure the children's safety. I preferred a rural setting, preferably with a lot of trees. On the other hand, we could not be too cut off. We needed to be within reach of doctors, stores, and a community to which the youngsters could be introduced as they were making progress.

The house I finally settled on was called Linwood. It was located at the end of a small road on the outskirts of the town of Ellicott City, in Maryland, about halfway between Washington and Baltimore. It came with a lot of land and was bordered by woods on three sides. The house had belonged to a family with a dozen children, so it was big enough for our purposes, but for a number of years it had stood empty and nothing had been done to it. It was structurally sound, but in every other way it was in terrible shape. The electrical system was antiquated to the point of being dangerous. Water came from a well in the yard, which was inadequately protected by a wooden cover and broke down at regular intervals, often helped along by children throwing twigs into the pump. There was central heating of sorts—hot air from an oil furnace entered some of the rooms by way of grates set in the floor—but most of the rooms only had open fireplaces.

I had purchased the property with a down payment of a few hundred dollars—some of it borrowed from friends, some contributed by the husband of a psychiatric consultant whom I had worked with at Children's House and who became our first medical director. I put all the money I had in the world into the project, without giving too much thought to the future. When I told Dr. Kanner what I had done he shook his head and said "Jeannie, Jeannie, you are putting your career on the line." But he promised his support, and no one was more delighted than he when Linwood flourished.

During the first months, the children could not live in, because we lacked any but the most primitive furnishings—improvising tables and shelves from orange crates, for example. Friends and the children's parents also chipped in, but it wasn't until we got a number of old hospital beds from an institution that we were able to keep the children in residence. It took a lot of creativity and improvisation to keep us going, but as people in the community began to hear about Linwood, they started visiting and we began to receive small monetary contributions as well as sorely needed things like drinking glasses and dishes.

The lack of funds meant that we could only bring the house up to required standards very slowly. For the longest time we lived dangerously close to disaster. To this day I do not know how we managed to stay open. We were in every possible violation of every imaginable building and fire code. The authorities had told me that they could close us down at any time, but our obvious attempts to take care of the worst hazards and my promises of continued improvements seemed to appease them somehow. The inspectors who came out looked around in total disbelief, scratched their heads—and left.

The first thing I did was to board up most of the open fireplaces and to block the large floor vents covered with grates. It would have been all too easy and tempting for our children to pry them up and fall straight down into the basement. All we could afford to get us through the first winter was a large Franklin stove that had to be fed with coal. The coal was delivered through a chute into the basement and had to be carried up one, two, and three flights of stairs in small buckets. It took fifteen buckets to fill the Franklin stove alone. In the kitchen, we had a small woodstove that we also cooked on. During the day Caesar, our handyman, looked after the fires, but he left at three o'clock to drive the children back to Washington. Then I had to take over, making sure that the stove got stoked every four hours, even during the night. Before it could be refilled, the old ashes had to be emptied out—no small task, since the cheap coal that we could afford contained a large quantity of stones.

One night, after I had finally gone to bed, the house started to get colder and colder. I discovered that the fire in the big stove had gone out because I had crammed too much coal into it. I felt like crying. I had to empty out all the coal and ashes and start all over again before I could return to bed. It became clear that we could not continue this way, especially once the children were going to be in residence and more of the rooms would need to be heated. Luckily, we got a donation large enough that we could afford to have a proper heating system installed. In the second winter we enjoyed the luxury of oil-fueled baseboard heat, and the last of the fireplaces were boarded up.

Keeping the house warm and clean were not the only challenges we faced during the early months and years. Everybody helped out where help was most urgently needed. Visitors might at one time find me covered in coal dust or ashes from wrestling with the Franklin stove, at another with a plunger in my hand, trying to unclog a toilet. One day the doorbell rang after the children had left, when I was cleaning our one bathroom. I ran down and opened the door and someone asked for the director. There I was, with an apron on and a toilet brush in my hand, and I said, "That's me."

Depending on the weather, staff and children might all be milling around in the one warm room in what must appear to the uninitiated as utter chaos, or the children might be roaming the yard, frequently watching with interest as I climbed yet again down into the well to clean out the pump and try to start it up again. The first summer, the water level became lower and lower, and finally the well went dry altogether. This meant that we had to borrow water from our neighbors or fetch it from a creek half a mile away.

Money, or rather the lack of it, was the refrain to all our activities and put restrictions on what we were able to do. But we had a very active and dedicated board with members who spread the word about Linwood within the community, and I also talked to every group I could think of. Several of them became interested in our work and would come for a guided tour, often leaving more perplexed than enlightened. They didn't always seem convinced that we knew what we were doing, but fortunately for us they were usually impressed enough to make a financial contribution anyhow.

Still, we didn't have any money to spare for major purchases. The cost for the children's stay had to be borne by the parents, because at that time this kind of special education was not covered by insurance. I tried to keep the fees as low as I could, which meant that they just about covered the price of food, utilities, and other unavoidable expenses. My devoted staff worked for a pittance, and for the first year we were in operation I could not afford to allot myself a salary. I did not mind. I have never worried about money, and my basic needs were taken care of. I took my meals with the children and at first also lived at Linwood, where I had a small room to myself on the third floor. But some expenses were unavoidable. Most of our children initially came from Washington and had to commute to Linwood every day. We had to make some provisions for transporting them.

We put an ad in the paper to see whether anybody might have a car they would be willing to donate to us, and sure enough, we got an answer. The car we were offered was a big black contraption that frankly looked like a hearse. It was extremely temperamental and rarely went more than a few miles without stopping. Fortunately, Caesar turned out to be as handy with engines as he was with everything else, but every day I listened for the "chug-chug" coming up the road, never knowing whether the car would stall once again before turning into our driveway. During one memorable trip, the engine gave out ten times between Washington and Linwood. Worse even than the unreliable engine was the fact that the doors didn't lock. We used rope to hold shut the doors, grasping them in one hand while holding on to the children with the other. It became obvious that we had to give up on the limousine. When we told the man who had given it to us, he was very surprised. He insisted that it should be in excellent condition, since for the last fifteen years it had been used in a high school shop by students learning basic mechanics!

The initial staff consisted of Miss Becky, a young aide from Children's House who seemed to have an instinctive understanding of how to work with our children; Caesar, who had worked as a janitor at Children's House and became our indispensable handyman and chauffeur; and me. In addition, three women from Ellicott City took turns helping with the many different household duties: cooking, cleaning, and acting as practical nurses when necessary and, later, occasionally taking over night duty.

I was always on duty during the first months. I worked with the children and I helped out in the kitchen or with the cleaning or acted as a nurse. I also kept the books and did small repairs. I lived, ate, slept, and breathed Linwood. I could never get away from it, and the strain was beginning to tell. After about six months a small cottage next to Linwood became available, and the board rented it for me. I stayed in that cottage for twenty years.

Once we had fixed up the house to make it reasonably safe and comfortable and had acquired some furniture, we were ready to operate as a residential center. We started with ten children. Since we did not yet have a regular night staff and I didn't know what was going to happen, I was, naturally, on duty. It turned out to be a very long night indeed. The children were completely uninterested in going to bed.

Rather than stage a futile struggle, I kept them out in the yard to see what would happen. They played in the sandbox, sat on the grass, or climbed on the equipment. Ten o'clock came, then eleven o'clock. I sat and watched. The children were wide awake. Midnight passed, and still they seemed to be going strong. Then the one sitting on top of the swing set fell asleep. We took him down and put him to bed. One after the other the children started to droop and were carried in. But I sat up for the rest of the night to make sure they stayed put. Later I moved a cot to the foot of the stairs to make sure that none of the children would escape from the two rooms on the second floor we had converted to dormitories. There were too many ways they could get into trouble, and they often did so, even though we watched them closely.

With the children in need of supervision day and night, it was necessary to hire additional staff. I engaged a live-in housemother, a practical nurse, and a teacher. By that time I had officially moved into the cottage, but as long as the children were in residence I was rarely completely off duty. Usually the children went home for the weekend, but one unforgettable weekend during our second winter, our housemother and I were left with five youngsters.

One of them was sick with a high fever. All of them were among our most difficult children. Without warning, it started to snow. The flurries quickly turned into a blizzard, and within a very short time the wet snow started to bring down branches from the big trees lining the driveway and the road, and with them went the electric lines, so that we were without light or heat. As soon as I realized what was happening I called our medical director, who lived in Washington, to tell her of my fear of getting cut off and to ask for advice and help. The storm was apparently localized and it was only snowing lightly in Washington, so she must have thought that I was overreacting and did not take my concerns very seriously. Before I could figure out who else I could call, the telephone went dead.

It continued to snow. Every so often we could hear the crack of a breaking tree limb reverberating like a gunshot through the eerie quiet of the falling snow. Then the electrical lines snapped in a shower of sparks and blue flickering lights that resembled northern lights. There was nothing we could do. The downed lines made it too dangerous to leave the house.

With no heat, the house quickly grew cold. I gathered all the children in one room, where I had managed to pry the boards off the fireplace. With some paper and coal, I started a small fire and over it managed to heat some of our store of canned foods in assorted pots and pans from the kitchen. As it got dark, the fire also provided us with some light. The children watched my attempts at assembling some kind of meal with interest, but they insisted that supper had to be eaten in the dining room. I persuaded them that this was not really supper but a picnic, like the ones we had when we went on outings in a nearby state park.

Since this was the only room with any heat, I brought down the children's bedding and arranged it as close to the fire as was safe. The hallway to the bathroom was lit by a candle stub safely out of reach of the children. They had rarely seen lighted candles except on some special, festive occasion, and one child sang "Happy Birthday" every time he had to go to the bathroom.

The night was absolute murder. The children slept only fitfully, and I had to stay up to feed the fire and to make sure none of them got too close to it or wandered off. I also had to look after the sick child. The next morning there was ice and snow as far as we could see. I opened another batch of cans. The children insisted on having breakfast downstairs. Again, I suggested that this was a picnic, but I was firmly corrected: "No breakfast picnic. Only supper picnic."

The sick child was getting worse, and our store of food and fuel was limited. Something had to be done. One of our intrepid employees, a practical nurse–helper from Ellicott City, had managed to fight her way through the snowdrifts to offer some relief. I decided to leave the children in her care and try to get help. I gave her all the cookies and candy I could find and told her to do whatever she needed to keep the children in the one warm room. Then the housemother and I started to clear off her car and shovel out enough of the drive to point the car in the right direction. With her steering the car and with me continuing to clear away the worst snowdrifts and other obstacles along the way, we managed to inch down the road, skirting the fallen wires, until we found a working phone.

After much calling around, I located the medical director at her hairdresser. She was not pleased to be called to the phone. I described our predicament—the lack of heat, electricity, and food—and told her about the sick child in urgent need of medical attention.

She listened to my tales of woe and then told me somewhat curtly, "You best put a white flag on the roof."

I was so stunned by this advice that all I managed to say was "Where?"

"On the little tower, of course," came the impatient reply.

The woman was obviously serious. I didn't have the energy to ask her how she proposed I reach the top of the roof or, even if I managed such a feat, who she thought would be likely to see a white flag in the expanse of whiteness surrounding us. All I could do was to hang up. With nothing accomplished, we returned to our charges.

In the meantime, the parents of one of our children had heard about the freak storm that had apparently only affected a relatively small area. They had tried to call Linwood and, getting no answer, had contacted the police in Ellicott City. The person they spoke to could not get through to Linwood on the phone either but had reassured the parents by telling them that we had probably already been evacuated. But the police had their hands full digging out the homes of elderly citizens. They knew that Linwood was a solid building that was unlikely to collapse, so it was not on their priority list. They may also have thought that the building was empty for the weekend. In any case, we spent another day holed up in our one room with increasingly restless children and the attraction of picnics fading fast.

I was getting pretty desperate. We faced another night of dark and cold and I was exhausted. It was late, the children had finally settled down, and I was looking out into the pitch-black night when all of a sudden I saw two lights approaching from the road. They turned out to be the headlights of a huge vehicle that slowly churned up our drive. When it finally came to a stop in front of the house, some men in army uniforms jumped out, and one of them, a very young soldier, proudly announced: "We have come to save you!"

And save us they did. Out of pure desperation and after consultation with the nurse, I had ended up giving the children a mild sedative to calm them down. They were either asleep or very drowsy when the soldiers wrapped them in blankets and carried them to the truck. One of the children, surveying the scene, mumbled sleepily, "Now we belong to the army." But they put up no resistance to the whole adventure.

I was told that we would be taken to Ellicott City, where we would occupy the officers' quarters of the National Guard unit to which our "saviors" belonged. Knowing the havoc our children could create within minutes, I was somewhat apprehensive about what might happen to those accommodations, but the first thing was to get them someplace warm and safe. On the way, we passed a doctor's house and stopped there to consult him about our sick child. He diagnosed pneumonia, prescribed penicillin, and offered to put up the child and our nurse for the rest of the night. We left them there and then continued on to the barracks.

The officers' quarters were furnished very nicely, with tables, chairs, cots, and lamps, and anything else we could possibly need. I thanked the officer on duty for making us so comfortable but told him that our youngsters would destroy these beautiful things in no time, so the rooms would have to be emptied of everything but the bare essentials. We cleared out anything I thought might tempt the children. What I couldn't do anything about were the bathrooms. One of the boys had a passion for faucets. He loved to take them apart and could do so with amazing skill and speed. When he saw the shower room with at least ten showers in them, he must have thought he had gone to heaven. Before he could be stopped, he had disassembled most of the fixtures.

Finally I had everyone settled down. I told the housemother to go to bed, too, that I would sit up for the rest of the night. Just as things were quieting down, I heard singing coming down the hallway and in marched a young officer who was clearly happily inebriated. He was past noticing anything, least of all that the room was occupied, but marched straight toward one of the cots and prepared to lie down on it. I had some trouble getting through to him but finally managed to steer him toward one of the back rooms. He took the whole thing with good humor and disappeared.

The poor housemother, who was a very proper and demure lady, had lain there through the whole incident with the covers pulled up over her head, terrified of this noisy male intrusion. After a while she emerged again and decided to take a shower before going to sleep. She was only halfway through when our officer reappeared. He had to go to the bathroom, and his need obviously admitted of no delay. My poor friend shot out of the shower wrapped in all the towels she could find, dove under the covers, and was not seen for the rest of the night.

I sat up through my second night with the restless children, and by the time the bus came to take them to Washington and their parents, I was totally exhausted. I went on the bus with them and made sure they were all delivered safely. I did not know where to go myself. Even if I could have organized transportation, I could not go back to Linwood until the basic services were restored. I had hardly any money on me, so I finally asked to be dropped off at the house of the medical director, where I hoped to get a badly needed shower and some sleep. Instead, she decided to call a meeting to discuss the situation. I pointed out to her that I had not been out of my clothes in over forty-eight hours. When she insisted on holding a meeting, I left and went to the YWCA.

I found out later that she had taken my plea for help more seriously than I had thought, but her contribution had consisted of contacting some people in Baltimore to arrange for a food drop from a helicopter. It obviously never occurred to her to think about how we could have reached the dropped food through the waist-high snow or, having reached it, how we would have cooked it without electricity and how we could have kept the children safe and warm without light or heat.

As soon as the roads were safe I returned to my cottage, where I had a working fireplace and a gas stove. The son of one of our employees waded up the road every day or so and deposited some milk and other things near the driveway, so I only had a short way to go to retrieve it. It took two weeks for the electrical lines to be repaired and the roads opened; then we were able to turn the heating system on again and were back in business.

WE WERE SCRAPING BY NOW, but for many years we were so chronically short of funds that I had to moonlight to bring in extra cash. Fortunately, the director of a nearby private psychiatric hospital was happy to have me provide therapy for some of his more difficult adolescents. I had occasionally worked with him while I was still at Children's House, so he knew and trusted me. The memory of some of the youngsters I saw there stayed with me.

I especially remember an eighteen-year-old schizophrenic girl who had been institutionalized for several years. She had had a psychotic break when her father, with whom she had been exceptionally close, remarried and had another child. She had to be kept in an empty room by herself because she not only refused to communicate or keep herself clean, but smeared feces all over the walls and the floor. She also spat all over everything.

When I was let into her room I saw a naked girl crouching on a mattress on the floor, her face hidden behind a curtain of long, tangled hair. The walls were covered with spit and drawings and writing executed with feces. I had been warned about going into her room by myself, because she was known to be aggressive at times.

I asked that a chair be placed inside the door for me and then introduced myself to her. She did not acknowledge the introduction, nor did she show any awareness of my presence. I sat on the chair, not saying anything. She continued her spitting, but somehow I escaped being doused. After about half an hour I left, telling her that I would come back to see her. I came back the next day and the next, and the same thing happened every time. She continued crouching on her mattress in her filth, hiding behind her hair and spitting.

This went on for several weeks. I began to get very tired of sitting in this disgusting room with its smell of excrement. I knew that it would not be helpful to let myself get to the point where I would be so fed up with it that I might get upset at the girl. The time had come to issue an ultimatum. I was pretty sure that I could risk it, because I had noticed that, while she never acknowledged my presence, she never actually spat on me. She left a clearly defined clean space around me, and that made me think that she not only was aware of my presence but actually welcomed it.

So, one day, I came in, sat down as usual, and said, "You know, I have to tell you something. It stinks in here. It is filthy, you are dirty, your hair is a mess, I have never seen your face. I have had enough of this. If you want me to continue to see you, you'll come out and take a bath and get dressed. Otherwise, I will leave, because it is disgusting in here."

For the first time, she parted her hair and peered out at me. Then she stood up and gestured that she was ready to be taken out of the room.

I stationed myself outside the half-open door of the bathroom and told her that once she had taken a bath, I would come in and help her with her hair. So that's what we did. Then she got dressed and we went for a little walk in the grounds.

I held on to her arm and suddenly she burst out, "Why are you holding on to me? Are you afraid?"

I said, "Well, first of all, I thought that perhaps by now we have become kind of friends, but secondly, I think that you are planning to run and I don't want to have to run after you. Also, if you did run, we couldn't go out anymore."

She looked at me with a frown on her face. I had been right, but she did not attempt to run.

This marked the breakthrough. Although she was still spitting and smearing, she agreed to take a bath whenever I came to see her. After a few days of this, I told her "Tomorrow, I will come at such and such a time, and by that time you will have had your bath and be dressed"— and she was.

After a while she asked whether she could come to my apartment. I agreed, and got friends to provide the transportation. She was still spitting all the time, however, so as she entered the car I told her "This is not my car. If it was my car, I don't know what I would do, but this is the car of friends, and they are kind enough to help me so you can come to my apartment, so spitting is out." She was able to keep from spitting during the whole trip.

When we got to my cottage she immediately started to spit again. I had a very nice parquet floor, so I said, "Wait a moment. I have told you that if it was my place, it would be different, but I have a special place for spitting, and that is the bathroom. You can spit all you want to in there, but there are limits at my house." So she went into the bathroom and did an awful lot of spitting.

After a while I brought in a bucket and said, "Now we will clean it up." She did so without protest. I prepared dinner and she ate it with fork and knife, although at the hospital she was only given a spoon, because she was still occasionally aggressive.

I invited her to spend the night, but she reminded me that she wet the bed. I told her that I was aware of that and had prepared for it, that I had plenty of sheets and had also covered the mattress. She gave me a look that seemed to say "Am I ever going to get you?"

As she went to bed, I saw that she was getting ready to have a bowel movement right then and there. I said: "Sorry. You told me about wetting the bed, and that's OK, but bowel movements are done in the bathroom."

She went into the bathroom, and when I went in to check I saw that she had defecated in the bathtub. I said, "Fine. Now let's get this taken care of properly." I gave her paper to put the stools in the toilet with and brought some Clorox bleach and water and had her clean out the tub. I had no problems after that. She knew I meant business, she knew the limits, and she also knew that she would never come back if she did not respect them.

I had her back at my house several times after that with no problems at all. We also went to the movies after some further improvements, and later still she was even able to go by herself. But she was still a very sick girl. After about a year and a half, her father, who lived in Florida, decided to pull her out of treatment and have her live in Florida. He had not discussed this plan with the psychiatrist or with me. When her father came to pick her up, the director thought that I had made these arrangements with him. The girl apparently thought so, too. She must have felt terribly betrayed by me for letting her go before she was ready. I will never forget the look in her eyes, as if I had abandoned her. But there was nothing I could do. I heard later that her father had promised to set her up in an apartment of her own but instead had quickly put her into another institution near him when he saw that she was not able to function independently yet.

While this was a psychotic youngster, the work with her was in many ways no different from work with Lee or with the children at Linwood. I have never been interested in labels. I have always approached every individual I have worked with without thinking about either diagnosis or prognosis, and I have used whatever they have given me to motivate them to change and grow at whatever pace they were ready for.

I took on other outside consulting work as well, and by the end of our third year in operation at Linwood things had begun to stabilize somewhat and the results of our work were so encouraging that it was clear that we were here to stay.

I DON'T KNOW WHEN I began to realize that the term *autism* might apply to my group at Children's House and our children at Linwood. I was in contact with Dr. Kanner because of Lee and some of the other children he had supervised at Children's House. By the time I started Linwood, we had become friends.

Dr. Kanner approved of what I was doing and seemed to especially like that I never used jargon or somebody else's techniques. He introduced me to a lot of professionals in the field, and I frequently was a guest at his house. Dr. Kanner never interfered with the way someone else approached a case, nor did he give direct advice. He mostly just shared with you what he saw, and left you to use that any way it made sense to you. He did not theorize, and if he ever talked to me directly about autism, I do not remember it. I learned about it later by reading about it. But we talked a great deal about the children I worked with, and in that way I discovered that my group was very much like the children he was seeing, all of whom showed remarkably similar behaviors, rarely seen in this combination in other youngsters.

The most striking and telling of these behaviors was the children's inability to relate. They shied away from contact or ignored it, reacting with varying degrees of protest to intrusions into their personal space or treating other people merely as objects—at most using an available hand as a tool to get what they wanted. Along with this went a lack of communication, either a total absence of language or meaningless words and phrases used indiscriminately. Some children had echolalia, repeating anything and everything they heard but without knowing what it meant and without being able to use their extensive vocabulary appropriately.

Most of the children engaged in some kind of compulsive behaviors related to certain objects or taking the form of obsessive rituals that they performed at certain times or in certain situations and to which they clung with single-minded persistence. When their favorite objects were removed or they were interrupted in their compulsive activities, they showed great distress, often expressed in severe temper tantrums, which in extreme cases could include self-aggressive behaviors.

Another common characteristic was the children's reaction to change. They noticed and resisted the slightest change in their environment or routine, and even within a known environment often staked out a small space within which they seemed to feel safe and from which they could be coaxed only slowly and gradually. This resistance to change also made it difficult for them to learn or to expand their activities in any way. They often appeared fixated on one aspect of the environment: certain numbers, number or letter combinations, shapes, dates, the weather, or a particular food, leading to feeding problems. Many of the children at one time or another also exhibited irrational fears.

Because of the lack of communication and the varying degrees of verbal delays, it was often impossible to assess their intellectual potential. By conventional standards all of them would have been diagnosed as retarded, some to a significant extent, and despite gradual and often striking improvements in their ability to relate and communicate and a reduction in compulsive behaviors, most of them never did progress beyond a special-education level.

However, I also worked with a number of highly intelligent children, especially during the early years, when the public schools did not yet have specialized programs for children with these kinds of problems. After graduating from Linwood, these youngsters went on to regular schools and in some cases got advanced degrees. Mostly they chose careers that involved work in an inanimate, orderly environment with little need for human interactions, which continued to be difficult for them.

Even the most intelligent autistic youngsters displayed a telling cognitive characteristic. They were unable to think at any but a concrete level. They took everything that was said absolutely literally and therefore could not understand verbal puns or metaphors and could not use them themselves. They lacked the ability to speculate and fantasize, which was also evident in their play. They could imitate, but not act "as if," so there was hardly any "pretend play," such as playing "house." Most of our children actively disliked dolls, and doll play, if it occurred at all, was always a sign of significant progress.

Because of their literalness, these children were locked into the world as it could be seen, touched, tasted, felt, and heard. They could not escape these limitations and therefore had a hard time recognizing and dealing with such intangibles as feelings. Lee, for example, had to translate his distress caused by jealousy into a physical sensation he was familiar with. They also lacked a sense of humor, since that requires one to be able to step outside a situation and see it, or oneself, in a different, unexpected, or absurd light.

Two of the most important ingredients in working with these children are patience and the ability to give without expecting anything back. Change comes very slowly and the children are emotionally closed off, so they do not become attached in ways that gratify the caretaker's emotional needs. For anyone who approaches work with autistic children with an unconscious agenda of wanting to "feel good by doing good," this work ends up to be very frustrating.

Autistic children are much more likely to become attached to the house, the yard, a tree, or another specific object in their environment than to the caretakers who have worked and lived with them, sometimes for years. I remember one youngster who wanted to visit Linwood several years after he had left us. He wrote to me saying something like "Dear Miss Simons, if you are still alive, I will come to see you, if not I will come anyway to see the house."

In this respect, I seem to have a distinct advantage over other people. Being autistic myself, I have a need for emotional distance that makes it easier for me to see and respond to the needs of others without becoming invested in having a child become dependent on me or "repay" my commitment to him by being grateful or attached to me.

As I mentioned in the preface, Jeanne and I often talked about this fundamental difference between her and most other therapists. Jeanne thought her lack of ego in the Freudian sense not only gave her a clearer view of the children she worked with but also allowed her to remain nonjudgmental, unaffected by the patient's reaction or non-reaction and even abuse of her. She did set limits on physical abuse, if only because she knew her own limitations in staying in a situation where she got hurt.

One of her favorite stories was of a boy she had treated at Linwood who visited her as an adult. He reminded her of how she had set limits on his abusive behavior by telling him, "If you kick me with your shoes on, it will hurt me and I will get angry, but if you kick me in your socks, it will be all right." He added, "So you let me kick you till I didn't have to do it anymore."

Possibly because of the constant vigilance demanded by my own vulnerability, I have become an excellent observer of others and can gauge when a person is ready for change and the time for an intervention has come. I am convinced that this, as much as anything, is responsible for my success in working with even the most difficult and seemingly inaccessible children and is the basis of the "intuition" that I have often been credited with.

Knowledge of a particular child, based on close and patient observation, usually yields some clues as to the type of intervention that is likely to be the most successful at any given time. I believe that this "intuition" is shared by most good therapists and that it can be learned to some extent, though I do seem to have an advantage over other people.

Lee and Martin and the other children who made up the initial group at Children's House and at Linwood displayed many if not all of the characteristics described above, as I realized once I had begun to study the phenomenon. But while I learned a lot about autistic symptoms and behaviors from Dr. Kanner and from my own observations, I could not, at first, find many people who were working specifically with this type of population. Some who claimed to treat autistic children, like Bettelheim at his Orthogenic School in Chicago, were actually dealing with a mixed population that included a large number of psychotic children.

Long after Dr. Kanner had clarified his initial concept of "refrigerator parents" as the possible cause of autistic symptoms, Bettelheim persistently claimed that the disorder was caused by cold, rejecting, incapable, and neglectful mothers. Knowing the extreme length of self-sacrifice many of the parents went to, their commitment to their children, and their often frustrating search for help, I found Bettelheim's views to be cruel and unhelpful, to say the least.

In my search in the literature and around the country, I found other professionals who approached the treatment of children with autistic characteristics not from a psychoanalytic perspective, like Bettelheim, but from a purely behavioral one. They focused on behavior they wanted the children to develop, such as eye contact or speech, and rewarded every manifestation of this, usually by giving the children some food. Undesirable behaviors, compulsions, self-aggression, etcetera, on the other hand, were punished to eventually get rid of them. This punishment was not always very subtle or humane. In one unforgettable institution I visited, I remember the staff using electric cattle prods to extinguish undesirable behaviors.

Sometime during the first two years Linwood was in operation, I heard about this marvelous treatment center for autistic children near Washington. I was eager to visit it, but when I investigated, I discovered that the institution talked about was—Linwood. Word about our work had apparently spread without my even being aware of the reputation we were acquiring in the professional community.

IN 1967, THERE WAS AN EPIDEMIC of the Asian flu. I decided to get inoculated but may already have been incubating the illness when I got the shot. In any case, I became seriously ill, with symptoms reminiscent of the encephalitis I contracted when I was seventeen. I had seizures again and was paralyzed, this time on my right side. The illness was diagnosed as a viral brain infection and I was hospitalized at the Johns Hopkins Hospital for six weeks.

I had to learn to walk all over again, and at first was also unable to write. Since my brain did not seem able to send messages to my right leg, I had to look at my foot and touch my leg to move it. I practiced endlessly, supporting myself between two bookcases. As my leg slowly got stronger I regained some feeling in it so that I was able to move it without the help of touch and sight. But for months, I had to use a cane to walk.

I also devised my own physical therapy to relearn writing. Even after I had some strength back in my arm and hand, I had trouble with small-muscle coordination and could not control my hand and fingers enough to form small letters or write in a straight line. I used two large rulers to define the space within which to practice my script and to help me stop when I reached the top or bottom of a letter. It took me many months before I could walk again independently. Writing without props took even longer.

AS MORE RESEARCH FOCUSED on this "new" disorder, more and better treatment approaches and facilities opened, with approaches that were more similar to the one that guided my own work, such as the work done by Dr. Eric Schopler at the University of North Carolina at Chapel Hill, and at the Center for Autistic Children in Philadelphia, headed by Dr. Bertram Ruttenberg. Autistic behavior was being understood as part of a continuum of seriously disabling behaviors that need not prevent youngsters from becoming socially integrated and participating in life in many important ways, if they got the right kind of help early on.

Funding remained a problem for the next twenty years, until the passage of Public Law Number 94-142 in 1975, which mandated the use of public funds for the education of children with special educational needs. Before then, we scrounged for funds from every source. Some came from social agencies, most from generous citizens impressed by our work. We also got the US Department of Health, Education, and Welfare to fund a research project by Dr. Charles Ferster, a behavioral psychologist from the Institute of Behavioral Research then located in Silver Spring, Maryland. He designed a study in which he tested some of his ideas on operant conditioning on our children. He worked at Linwood from 1966 to 1969, and despite our very different ways of thinking about treatment, we learned a lot from each other and became good friends. We stayed in touch even after his work at Linwood was concluded. His death struck me as a great loss, because with him I got a little bit of an idea what it might feel like to have a relationship.

Concurrent with Dr. Ferster's work, Dr. Kanner engaged in an outcome study with me at Linwood in which he examined thirty-four children with varying diagnoses in 1966. He did follow-ups in 1968 and again in 1973.

As our work became better known in the professional community, our number of children gradually increased from the original ten to around thirty. In 1973, when the original building no longer met changing fire and health standards, it was renovated and a separate dormitory was added. By that time we also had redesigned our program, continuing with a residential component, but adding two types of day programs, one coinciding with the regular school day, the other extending into the evening.

As time went on, one of my biggest concerns was what would happen to Linwood once I retired. If my work had any value beyond my own immediate contributions, it would survive me. If others could not duplicate it, I was nothing more than an interesting phenomenon, a freak. So it was very important to me that people came to Linwood to be trained, to take what they learned there and apply it to their own work. We had people from Japan, Holland, France, Germany, and Ireland pass through Linwood at varying times. I was also glad to cooperate with professionals in other institutions in America and abroad, and for many years consulted with a psychiatrist in France whenever I was in Europe. More recently, I have lectured and consulted in Switzerland, Greece, Japan, and Mexico.

But most important to me is and was Linwood and its children. I carefully selected and trained the staff and gave a lot of thought to my successors. Once I retired, I wanted to do so completely, entrusting Linwood to others and let them run it the way they saw fit, even if they did things their own way. I would be there to be consulted and even continue to work with some of the children, but I did not want to second-guess anybody or have them look at me forever for guidance.

As it happened, I was fortunate to find several especially gifted young people who worked with me until they were able to take over various components of the program on their own. Their Linwood is no longer the Linwood I began. The program has expanded beyond my wildest expectations. It now serves not only children but also adolescents, and since 1988 there is a new component: sheltered housing for adults who have graduated from our program. In addition to the various treatment groups, there is an adapted school program for the more advanced children, there is vocational training for the adolescents, and there is supervision for young adults who go to jobs in the community.

Linwood is evolving like any living organism, and its vitality makes me feel very rich indeed.

Anyone reading this account, especially the stories from Linwood's early days, meets a woman of vison, determination, and seemingly inexhaustible energy. Yet at the time Jeanne established her program for the most difficult children imaginable and ran it with a skeleton staff in a house that lacked the most basic amenities, she was already forty-five years old.

Who am I?
The search for self

13

I took every opportunity to expand my knowledge of autism and contacts among those who studied and treated autistic children, but despite my growing understanding of autism and the experience I gained in working with this special group of children, I had not made the connection to my own experiences and behaviors as a child and young adult.

I had never been self-reflective and had never compared myself to others. And I had learned very early to avoid situations that were dangerous for me or to build walls against them. But I lacked an accurate self-image. To this day, when I am in my seventies, I am still trying to define the different parts of myself and discover who I am. Although I have good drawing ability, for example, and have done a number of portraits in pastels—my favorite medium—I can still not draw myself. If pressed to produce a self-portrait, I could only represent myself as a stick figure.

Then one day, after people started coming to Linwood from all over, in the early 1960s, somebody sort of jokingly said: "How can you understand the children the way you do? It is almost as if you were like that yourself, or as if you had some similar experiences." That innocent remark came like a shock to me, and yet it only confirmed some knowledge that must have been there all along. Once I made the connection, many things became clear to me. I now saw why I had had the strong conviction that I had found my life's work when I met Lee and the other youngsters at Children's House. It must have been at least partly due to my affinity with them. Just as I had recognized something in the parents I had evaluated during my in-

156

ternship without knowing what it was, so I recognized something in these children that mirrored my own experiences.

I, too, had to defend against relationships at an early age to protect myself against the emotions of those around me. I had gone into hiding, both literally, under a table, and metaphorically, by disappearing behind a sort of one-way mirror inside my head that shielded my own thoughts from the intrusion of others but allowed me to observe them from a safe distance. I, too, had suffered when faced with change. I, too, developed obsessive and ritualistic behaviors as safeguards against lurking threats, and I, too, took everything I was told very literally and lacked imagination, though not a sense of humor.

Once I realized that I was in fact autistic, I felt a great sense of relief. A secret that at some level I had always known existed was finally out in the open. I began to think about myself in a conscious way for the first time in my life. I had never indulged in self-reflection and had never thought about what I was doing or why, nor had I wondered about differences between myself and others, simply assuming and accepting that everybody lived life the way that seemed best for them.

I didn't feel special, yet people kept stressing how unusual I was. They especially harped on my "intuition," which they credited for my ability to select the right strategy for working with every child and to time interventions as if guided by some sixth sense. It seemed to me that they were making something that was very simple unnecessarily complicated, but perhaps they knew something I didn't. Perhaps I was different from others in a fundamental way.

I decided to try to find out all I could about this "intuition" and went looking for an interpreter, someone with specialized knowledge I could consult with. I thought that I would simply sit down with someone I trusted and be told what "intuition" was. That was really all I wanted. I got more than I bargained for. Before I knew it, I was engaged in the most painful and hazardous undertaking of my life.

As far back as I could remember, I had relied only on myself. I had instinctively done what was necessary to survive and function. Now I was seeking to understand some of the things I was curious about and turned to a psychiatrist I knew and considered a friend. But what started out as a seemingly simple quest for knowledge, fueled by my curiosity about the differences between my way of viewing my work and other people's interpretations of it, quickly turned into an intrusive, all-encompassing pursuit with no containment or respite.

Psychoanalysis focuses on the past, attempting to dislodge memories of traumatic events that may be repressed and that may fixate so much energy at an early developmental stage that normal emotional growth is prevented. For me, emotional memories are dangerous. The only way I had been able to survive was to hermetically seal off a great number of feelings and experiences before they became real. To try to recall or recreate them might destroy me.

I cannot recall another such period of misery, danger, and sheer torture in my life. I tried to comply with lying on a couch, but I became so anxious that I began to shake and refused to stay where I could be seen but could not see the other person. My inability to free associate was interpreted as resistance; the relative absence of emotions as denial; and my description of any lack of early relationships as intense, suppressed anger and hostility toward my parents, especially my father. Doggedly, the therapist preached her dogma and wrestled for my unconscious. She even started to associate for me.

Ever more bewildered, confused, and desperate, I tried to follow her lead and give her what she wanted, but I didn't know what that was. While I was slowly coming to the realization that something in me was indeed different from others, rather than getting a clearer picture of myself, I became more and more confused. What had seemed simple and ordinary became uncomfortable and strange. I did not recognize myself in the interpretations my therapist gave me, and could not identify with the feelings and motives she attributed to me. But whenever I did not accept one of her interpretations, she accused me of harboring suppressed hostility.

I had no emotional experience with relationships, so it was difficult to assess the one that was developing with my therapist. But I did know that instead of giving me useful insights, it weakened the survival instinct that had always stood me in good stead. Although I became more and more distressed, I could not extricate myself from the situation. I knew instinctively that I was being forced onto a wrong path, but initially I had trusted her, and later I felt trapped. I became more and more confused and desperate, and from my sense of helplessness there slowly grew anger, not the unconscious hostility the therapist was insisting I felt toward my parents, but an almost murderous rage toward her and her slow destruction of me.

One night, I had a strange dream. I saw myself climbing a high mountain. When I was at the top, I thought about throwing myself down and exploding into thousands of little fragments. These would drift down over the world, seeking out all the therapists who had ever done harm to people. The pieces would hurt anyone they touched, and the victims could not get rid of the pain because they didn't know where it came from. I remember feeling intense satisfaction, not only because of the power I had to punish them, but also because they could never escape the pain. But I hesitated, because I suddenly thought, still in my dream, "What if I were to hit a good therapist by mistake?" so I did not allow myself to jump off the mountain.

This dream frightened me a great deal and convinced me that I was on the road to self-destruction unless I broke away from my therapist. I remembered how as a young child I had realized that if I watched them closely, I would be able to understand people and help them. But at the same time, I had also instinctively known that if I could find a person's weak spot, it would be possible to use that knowledge to hurt someone. From that time on I daily said a little prayer: "Please, God, never let me harm anybody."

I know now that it is not only impossible but potentially extremely damaging to try to psychoanalyze an autistic person. It is easy to see why when one thinks about some of the basic concepts of Freudian analysis. One of the techniques psychoanalysis uses, for example, is free association and the interpretation of feelings as they express themselves symbolically in a stream of consciousness or in dreams. Autistic individuals deal in concrete facts, not symbols or metaphors. They have no imagination. If you try to free associate, you float in some in-between state, without anything to hold on to. It is very frightening.

Also, therapy takes place within a relationship. According to psychoanalytical theory, change comes about through transference and countertransference. The patient allocates various roles to the therapist and works through his feelings for the people the therapist thus comes to represent: father, mother, lover, sibling, boss, etcetera. The feelings coming from the patient evoke memories and feelings in the therapist which help him understand how others might be reacting to the patient. On the basis of this understanding he can provide feedback and interpretations to the patient, who may more easily be able to accept them from the therapist than from people with whom he is emotionally entangled in his private life.

It is easy to see that this is not a process that is applicable to the treatment of autistic people. It simply doesn't apply. There are no old relationships, so there is nothing to project. Countertransference— the therapist's own projection of feelings onto the patient—is something autistic people cannot deal with. These feelings pose a real threat and can do a lot of harm. Within whatever therapeutic relationship develops, the autistic person feels helpless and extremely vulnerable. And having to lie down makes you feel even more vulnerable, as does not being able to see the therapist. You give up the one-way mirror. You no longer look out, unseen and safe. Now you are the one who is exposed, and it is the other person who is invisible. That doesn't mean that you can't go back. But you have to stay on the firm ground of reality. The only way treatment is safe is to go from one fact to the next fact and try to make sense out of them.

When I told my therapist that I was stopping treatment, she tried to stall me. But once I understood how wrong and dangerous the whole thing was for me, I quickly regained enough self-confidence to resist her. Eventually I found a wonderful, skilled, and sensitive doctor who saw very quickly that he was dealing with an unusual case.

After the experience of the first therapeutic relationship, it took me a long time to develop a real sense of trust again. I was also handicapped by my previous therapist's insistence on the confidentiality of everything that transpired during our sessions. Since I took this quite literally, I was at first unable to share with my new therapist what had happened to me in my previous treatment and get his help in understanding it. But he must have sensed something of what I had been through anyway.

He also saw that I didn't fit into any of the usual categories. Although he was a Freudian analyst by training, he was willing and able to develop approaches that met my needs, rather than trying to treat me according to a set theory. He was also infinitely patient, never pushing me to go at a pace that was uncomfortable. Over the past twenty years, he has helped me to understand and accept my specific strengths and limitations and the ways I am like and unlike other people. I still don't have the complete picture. Sometimes I read something about myself and I think, "That's an interesting person," but I don't really connect it with myself.

THE WAY I PICTURE MYSELF is as having two sides. One I call my *left side*. It is the strong one. It is the one that comes from experience and is untouched by anything outside my own experience. Even as a child I had never adopted values or opinions simply because they were offered to me by some authority. I believed only what fit the facts as I experienced them myself and acted only on my own convictions. This was not because I thought I knew more than others, but because I didn't really have a choice. I could no more act against what felt was right than I could cheat or lie for my own advantage.

I never tried to impose my own values on others, and I have never judged them. If you judge someone, you become involved with that person to some extent. There is the beginning of a sort of relationship, a closeness that takes away some of your own freedom. Since I don't have relationships, I am also not dependent on what others think of me. When I was a child I tried to be inconspicuous, because to attract attention would make me vulnerable to intrusions that I then would have to expend a lot of energy to defend myself against. As an adult, especially in my professional capacity, I did whatever I knew was right, and people generally respected that.

I learned early on to conform, at least outwardly. I also learned not to ask questions, because I found they often embarrassed people or made them angry. When I had asked, it was always because I honestly had wanted to know, but my questions were sometimes taken for impertinence. One of the places this got me into trouble, for example, was catechism class, when I was only about eight years old and we were told the story of Solomon's judgment in the case of the child claimed by two mothers. We were told that the story showed that Solomon was the wisest man who had ever lived, though it wasn't clear to me whether this particular story was true or just a legend. I asked: "What if it was a legend? Then the man who made it up would be even wiser than Solomon." The priest was angry at my presumption, but I wasn't trying to be smart or rude. There was just something in me that needed to figure things out.

Though I have never let the opinions of others dictate to me, I am very much aware of them, and when I notice that something bothers someone, I don't do it anymore—not because I necessarily accept that I have done something wrong, but because I do not want to intentionally shock, anger, or upset anyone. You give something of yourself by being very honest, but if you are asked for advice or an opinion and your answer upsets the other person, you have to deal with their emotions. So you learn early to avoid such situations.

But even as a small child I could not simply take somebody's word for something. Although I consider myself religious, I have never believed everything the Church teaches, because some of the things we were told just didn't make sense to me. We were told, for example, that you had to go to church on Sundays. Not to do so was to commit a mortal sin. When I first heard this, I thought about it and I began to wonder: "Do they have a calendar in heaven? What if I went on Monday instead? Would they care, as long as I went once a week?" I asked the priest, and he got very angry. He must have thought I was trying to provoke him. But I tried it, and nothing happened, so I knew they were wrong.

I also couldn't accept that the Catholic faith was the only "true faith." Even when I was quite young, I knew that wasn't fair. How could there be a small group of people who were the chosen ones? We were not al-lowed to play in the street when we were schoolchildren, partly because that just wasn't proper for middle-class children in Holland at that time and partly because we were not supposed to associate with the Protes-tant children who lived nearby. I went along with this when I was young, but I never believed there was anything wrong with the Protestants, and as soon as I could get away with it without causing a stir, I started to as-sociate with them, with no harmful consequences to myself.

I never did anything just because I was told that it should be done that way. We were brought up with very definite, strict rules and strong values. If things were presented to me in a way that made sense to me I accepted them; if not I just filed them away in my mind and disre-garded them once I was on my own. In the same way today, whenever I read something or am told something, I take the essence of it and incorporate it into my own thinking, but it has to somehow fit in with what I have seen, heard, or experienced myself.

One of the things I did not question was what seemed the gener-ally accepted expectation that most girls would eventually get mar-ried and have a family. I had no clear idea of what it meant to be married. If I ever thought about it I pictured the marriage ceremony as I had seen it performed, but I didn't think beyond that. I knew all I needed to about sex and it didn't bother me. I don't think I would have had any problems with the physical side of marriage, but I had absolutely no concept of relationships, and I know now—and at some level probably knew then—that it would have been impossible for me to live with somebody in that kind of emotional intimacy. I could not have borne the constant, close association with another hu-man being, since a true two-way relationship is impossible for me. I would have felt smothered and panicky and would have had to with-draw from it.

I have never changed what I believe or am willing to do in order to attract, please, or impress another person. All the choices I make are my own. Nobody can break them down. That gives me great strength, and it is this strength that I think has seen me through the many difficulties and challenges of my life. Sometimes doing what feels right means questioning the conventional wisdom and even opposing it, as in my work at St. Vincentius. Sometimes it has forced me to take on a task that I very much wanted to avoid, such as accompanying Audrey to America. But I really don't have a choice.

I have never been aware of my achievements because I never thought of them as anything extraordinary. I didn't have to struggle to develop an effective way of working with people, for example. It is a gift. I just have it. I can't think of myself as special simply for having it, any more than I would think of someone as unusually intelligent because they knew what a lamp or a table was for. If I had to work hard to develop it, I might be able to say "OK, this adds something," and I might be proud of that, but I didn't. There is just something in me that is different. It may be that something is missing or that I have something others don't, but it makes me exquisitely sensitive to others while at the same time I can also be completely objective.

I call it a blessing and a curse. A curse, because you can't deny it. You have it and you have to work with it. I can't just say "Let it go." I have to use God-given things. Sometimes now I think: "Why me?" But for the longest time, I thought everyone had it. It was only in Boston College that it was pointed out to me that I was intelligent. And I accepted that. I can be very objective about myself. I can see the good things and talk about them. I don't see why you can't be honest about your accomplishments. But I have never gotten particular satisfaction from this. Awards and citations never meant much to me. It is not that I feel that I don't deserve them, I just don't know what they mean. They don't add anything to who I am.

Things are very simple for my left side. It is as straight as an arrow. It sees things without distortion. A Yes is a Yes and a No is a No. There is no in-between. My left side is strong and secure. Nothing has invaded it. I see clearly, I hear clearly. There is this terrific integrity and a sense of freedom, because my values are not attached to any particular theory.

But simple doesn't necessarily mean easy. I am very poor and very rich at the same time. I don't feel poor because I don't miss anything. You can't miss what you have never had. I have no regrets, but I have paid a price. At times what I did was not out of choice, not voluntary. I had to do what I did and I did the best I could and sometimes the price was very high.

I have recognized, without being able to put it into words, where the handicaps are and what my limits are. I never tried to go beyond them. I have always lived life to the fullest within these limits. As an adult I have always had a surplus of energy because I never wasted energy on unnecessary, fruitless things like anticipation, worries, or wishes.

In a way my lack of imagination, too, is strength. I don't worry about how things will be. I don't waste time thinking about things I can't do anything about. I deal with things as they occur. This is not courage. It is part of my concreteness. I cannot deal with abstractions. The anticipation of something joyful that doesn't happen is painful, not only because of the disappointment, but also because you feel bad that you wasted energy on it. There was an incident when I was a child of seven or eight, when I was looking forward to an outing. But it got rained out, and I cannot remember another thing I have allowed myself to look forward to since. In this instance, as in many other situations, I learned from a single experience rather than in the usual way of learning in little steps.

I am convinced that my autism is not innate but is the result of birth trauma, especially oxygen deprivation. Therefore, I think that I had the potential to relate normally. It was only through an accident of birth that I became so abnormally sensitive to the emotions engendered by human interactions that I couldn't tolerate them and had to close off from them. I had to protect myself against them or be destroyed, just like a person born without pigmentation has to avoid sunlight so as not to get burned. Since I could not tolerate or share emotions, I did not develop early two-way relationships, and so I have no model for what normal relationships are like. I don't know the most basic things about them—for example, what it feels like to love one's parents. I don't know what it is to be strongly attached to someone, to need someone or want someone to need me. These abilities have not developed through lack of use. I guess one could say that I became emotionally disabled. I call this my *right side*.

I had felt for a long time that there was something there. Ever since my encephalitis, I experienced myself as if I was composed of two halves. The one on the left was bathed in a bright light and was sharply defined, the one on the right was in darkness and nearly invisible. It was the left side through which I lived, and somehow it never allowed full awareness of the right side. Until I made a lot of progress in my therapy, I was convinced that the two sides could not function together, as if one had to die in order for the other to live. Now I can look at the right side and accept it as part of myself.

I had a dream some time ago that for me illustrates that acceptance. I saw myself standing tall and beautifully dressed in a blend of fall colors. Somebody handed me a baby, but as I reached for it, something like sand started to run out of it. Quickly the little body shrank, until all that remained was a curving white trace, the outline of half a baby, which I cradled gently in my arms. That baby, like the sickle of the new moon, is all that can be seen or that I can experience of my other half, but I have accepted it.

I am not afraid of my right side. Mostly I am curious about that shadowy part of myself, about which there is still much to learn. Another dream speaks to that curiosity: I am walking through a lovely countryside when I see the outlines of something that looks like a fortress, a big, black, seemingly impenetrable structure without doors or windows and resembling a castle. But just as I get close enough to reach out and touch it, the structure collapses, crumbling into a pile of dust. What remains are scattered pieces of solid rock, which I pick up and examine with great interest.

But while I accept my right side and continue to explore it, I also know that it has nothing to offer to the left side. It is too late to integrate the two sides. That would have had to start with early relationships. At this point, the two sides coexist and I feel safe in the knowledge that they don't have to be merged.

AS PART OF GETTING TO KNOW my right side and exploring what it is capable of, I have been trying to learn more about relationships. The only memory I have of anything I could call a relationship during my childhood was before I was four years old. I had a very bad case of scarlet fever and had to be isolated. I remember the doctor coming into my room through a French window. He was a gentle person and there was something coming from him that got through to me. It is the only memory I have of another person that carries a good feeling with it. I didn't resist it, and I remember it still. Perhaps I was too sick to keep my guard up. Perhaps it was because I sensed that he didn't want anything from me.

My brothers and sisters, my parents, visiting relatives, and friends were all only part of a certain environment and took their meaning from it. Once I lost the environment, I lost them too. In each new place there were new parents, new brothers and sisters, impermanent objects that were lost again any time we were separated or moved. At the time nobody seemed to notice anything strange about me, but my friends and family must have known too, without knowing, just as I did, that there was a difference.

Over the past years I have regularly returned to Holland and have picked up contacts from my youth. One of my friends said: "You know, nobody really knew what it was with you, what you were all about." They must have puzzled over me. I was well liked, but it seems there was something they could not penetrate, and they wondered.

When my brother Antoine and my sister Maria came to visit me in America on the occasion of the twenty-fifth anniversary of Linwood, and they saw our children, they said to each other: "You know, Jeanne was like some of these children her whole life." It was only at that point that Maria told me that somehow it was accepted in the family that I was different. I never played. I was considered the brainy one. But nobody seems to have noticed the extremes of my obsessive behavior, and only in retrospect did it seem to strike my sister that in a way it was as if I wasn't there at all.

Even today I cannot ask my family about myself or discuss the early years. But they see that my reactions are different from most people's. They say that I can take anything. They used to call me the "Rock of Gibraltar," and I get called by them whenever there is something really hard to deal with.

My parents died within one week of each other, both of cancer. I happened to be home for one of my regular fall visits. I had not realized how serious the situation was, since they had rarely been sick in their lives and were both in their eighties. I was very glad that I had had some time with them, but I never cried, I never grieved, I never feel I lost parents. I don't know what parents are. And yet, when I am in Holland and the family starts reminiscing—"Remember Mama, when she did this or that?"—I have to get away. I cut it off. I can't stand it.

Other people survive on emotional memories, but for me memories are dangerous. I feel that I could die from them. It is as if I lost things before I had them. If I had been able to relate I would have lost something, but I lost it although I had never really had it.

Over the past six or seven years, there have been a very few people with whom I have shared a closeness that I wasn't capable of earlier. So nowadays when I lose someone with whom I have been able to develop a little bit of a relationship, the loss is very big, because I lose all there is and all there might have been. And every little bit in a relationship that goes wrong hurts. You open yourself up, and it can be very painful.

I think that what helped me get through life is that I have a strong survival instinct. I was always aware of the temptation of giving up the struggle. It is a wonderful feeling to retreat where nothing can touch you. It's like turning off all the faucets. But you might also destroy something. You might lose the ability of ever getting back again. That would be a kind of death, and it goes against my nature to let something in me die.

It is also dangerous to let needs surface. They might drown all that was. I have learned to be content with what there is and with the many good concrete memories I have, mostly of experiences with nature. I cannot mourn what wasn't.

PERHAPS THERE ARE MANY PEOPLE who are simply considered different, or somewhat strange, who, like myself, have been able to adapt enough to get by and have even achieved some measure of success. I wonder.

And I still wonder who I am.

When Jeanne told me about the ordeal with the psychiatrist, I was hard pressed to understand why she had let herself be abused in this way. I knew her as an exquisitely sensitive and successful therapist, a well-trained professional, a person with laser vision as far as her patients were concerned, a survivor, and above all, a fierce advocate for her charges. Never in a million years would she have allowed anyone to do to a child in her care even a fraction of what she was subjected to by her therapist.

Jeanne was unable to explain why she had persisted with her treatment to the point where it almost destroyed her as a person. An explanation may perhaps be found both in the characteristics of people with autism spectrum disorder as they deal with social interactions and in Jeanne's own way of dealing with difficulties. As Lee and Martin and the other children's stories illustrate, individuals living with autism do not form typical relationship bonds. They therefore do not know from experience what to expect from a relationship and tend either to be withdrawn and unwilling to engage or naively ready to take people at face value. That Jeanne talked about her therapist as "a friend," even though this person failed her—one could even say abused her—is a case in hand.

Jeanne had many devoted friends and benefactors, but she knew friendship mostly by definition, just as she theoretically knew about concepts such as *transference* and *countertransference*. Only very late in life did she begin to get an inkling of what relationships were about, above and beyond shared activities and interests.

Conclusion

Jeanne Simons was a person living with autism. Autism was the warp, the underpinning of her life. But the woof, the thread that gave her personality its visible texture and color, was how she dealt with her condition, transforming what could have been disabling challenges into a gift that benefited children and parents the world over.

Jeanne was at once a complex and a very simple person. She was highly accomplished, with a realistic sense of her own accomplishments, yet diffident and modest almost to a fault. When she was "on," whether called upon to lecture or in congenial company, she was lively, impressive, and entertaining. When in repose or unobserved she often appeared inwardly focused or withdrawn.

Her interests were many: nature in all its forms, art, music, and literature. She spoke German, French, Dutch, and English and was widely traveled. She especially loved water and trees and surrounded herself with images of them, most of them of her own creation. She was a gifted artist, drawing in charcoal and developing her own technique of painting—a mix of watercolor and pastel. Because of her autism, she was unable to draw from nature or memory, instead using photographs as the concrete start for all her pictures. But despite her insistence that she was unable to do anything but copy a given image, her artistic talent and the use of the media she used transformed her pictures into true works of art.

During one of our last conversations, she acknowledged how glad she was to be out of the hospital—after repeated bouts of pneumonia—and back in her own room at the nursing center, surrounded by her own things. I commented that she had so many of her beautiful pictures to look at, and she asked me, "Do you have any?"

I reminded her that she had given me a number of her paintings, starting with a large picture of an autumnal tree after *The Hidden Child* had been published. Her expression became dreamy and she said with great feeling "I loved that tree." I suspect it was a real tree she was thinking of, one that at one or another difficult time in her life had provided her with the solace she was unable to get from human companionship. I also remembered that she had earlier told me how, to defend against the feeling of suffocating closeness to her mother evoked in her as a young child by the explanation of how babies were born, she had convinced herself that she had been born from a tree!

But above all, Jeanne was her work. Whenever we would get together, and after she had conscientiously and kindly asked after my family, the conversation quickly centered on things she had been pondering, something she wanted to share, something we might yet do, or projects she was in the middle of.

After her retirement she had more time to visit and consult with centers all over Europe, accept an invitation to Japan, and help establish and consult with centers in Mexico and Latin America, where a Spanish translation of *The Hidden Child* in 1992 (*El Nino Oculto*) had fueled a great deal of interest in her work. She even received an honorary doctorate from the University of Mexico.

She traveled well into her ninth decade without any thought to her own health or comfort. If some group or center invited her to come and consult with them, she went, mostly without getting paid for her services. When she returned, increasingly taking longer and longer to recover, I would sometimes express my concern about the health cost of these expeditions. She acknowledged that it was hard but made it clear that she would go as long as she was able to. "They need me, and I have to go," she said.

Jeanne also remained actively involved with Linwood in many ways until the last years of her long life, when her health began to fail. She ran an adolescent group for many years, met with parents, and participated in staff training. She was also on the board and continued to be an ambassador and fundraiser for Linwood.

Even toward the end of her life, when her short-term memory began to falter, she clearly recalled episodes of her earlier life and especially anything to do with Linwood, remembering with special delight the most difficult of the children who had passed through her care and whom she called "my naughty little angels."

One of the hardest things Jeanne did during the years I knew her was to move out of her beloved apartment, which bordered on a fringe of woods, into a retirement community. Having at that time no relatives living close by and being determined not to ever become a burden on friends or neighbors, she planned and made the move while still in good health. But she never truly recovered from wrenching herself from the environment that had defined her for close to twenty years. Even a couple of years after her move, surrounded by her own furniture, pictures, and mementoes, she would tell me, when I asked how she was, "You know, it is awfully hard. They are very nice here. There are many interesting people and they offer many activities. But I haven't really gotten used to it."

I visited Jeanne regularly and took her out to lunch—always at the same restaurant, where, if possible, we sat at the same table. When she became a resident in the assisted living part of her retirement community, she was only allowed to go out with a portable oxygen tank, which she hated. With a twinkle in her eyes, she would leave it behind in the car.

To the end she rebelled against the dependence of being tethered to an oxygen tank and the restrictions it and her increasing weakness imposed on her ability to leave the floor or even her bed. Even when she could no longer get around unassisted and had a broken arm from falling, she would sneak out of her bed as soon as she was on her own. She gleefully told me about her escapades, explaining that she was trying to do some knee bends and other exercises to regain her strength—

just as she had done so many time before in her life, when she had come back from life-threatening and debilitating illnesses.

During the last years of Jeanne's life, her short-term memory became increasingly unreliable and eventually failed her altogether. But she recognized staff, friends, and relatives and talked lucidly about the past right up to the end of her life. She was fortunate in having a niece who had relocated from Holland and lived nearby. This devoted relative and her partner saw to Jeanne's every need and toward the end were in daily contact with her and the staff who cared for her. Jeanne was very fond of her niece and became uncharacteristically dependent on her toward the end, frequently expressing her gratitude that she had her in her life. Perhaps she was able in a sort of second childhood to at last experience one close relationship.

On our last visit she told me that she had been thinking back to her earliest, preverbal memories (recounted at the beginning of this book), and again described them to me. Then this remarkable woman, gasping for breath, near death, and totally confused about everyday occurrences, who would forget that I had visited her half an hour after I left, told me, "You know, quite a few of the children I worked with had memories that went back very early, almost to birth. I wonder whether being able to remember that far back is a characteristic of autistic people. Nobody has written about this. It would be worth researching." (I am glad we included some of the children's very early memories in *The Hidden Child*.)

Jeanne died ten days later, in her ninety-sixth year, in 2005. The most moving contributions at the memorial service in her honor came from adults who had been among the first group of children at Linwood. Every one of them said that due to their experiences at Linwood they were able to support themselves, some of them in well-paid, responsible jobs. All of them attested that without Linwood, they would have seen out their lives in institutions.

Perhaps the most telling tribute was given by one of her former "naughty angels" who said, "Miss Simons never turned away any child."

JEANNE SIMONS TOUCHED and changed countless lives around the globe. She gave hope to desperate parents, support to professionals, and a better quality of life to any child who passed through her hands. This book, a look at autism from the inside out, is a testament to an indomitable spirit and the ability to overcome adversity. It rounds out Jeanne's legacy.

I hope that the book will be an inspiration to everyone who can now share in an unprecedented journey that spanned almost a century.

Epilogue
Linwood then and now

Jeanne Simons' Linwood Children's Center is no more, though the old mansion Jeanne bought in 1955 still stands.

It is an impressive stone house of locally quarried granite, with the older section believed to have been built shortly after the founding of Ellicott's Mills, possibly in the 1780s. The property Jeanne acquired was somewhat over four acres. The house, named "Linwood," was situated at the apex and overlooked a circular drive, meadows, and woods, with a small cottage—Jeanne's home for many years—as its nearest neighbor. There was ample space for a fenced-in play yard and, later, the addition of a separate dormitory building. Now the mansion stands empty, hemmed in by parking lots and nose to nose with a large, low, modern structure, its successor, the Linwood Center.

When Jeanne opened Linwood Children's Farm, later renamed the Linwood Children's Center, she saw it as a haven for children who were deemed uneducable. Early infantile autism (as it was then called), the disorder common to the first small group she had initially taught at a center in Washington, was not widely known at the time, and there were few if any dedicated programs for such children anywhere in the world. There were therefore also no specific treatment modalities to rely on for treating and educating the children, and Jeanne relied on her own training, insights, and instincts to fit her approach to the needs of individual children.

Because the children were severely symptomatic and often aggressive, they posed continuous challenges to their families, making a normal family life nearly impossible. Jeanne therefore initially conceived Linwood as a residential treatment center to offer intensive care to the children and, especially, relief to the afflicted parents.

As the center became known, not only throughout the region but the world, enrollment grew. With a number of children ready to be mainstreamed, it was converted into a day school, with an extended day option. At any one time, it served between twenty and thirty children in five classrooms on two levels, while the administrative offices were tucked in under the eaves on the third floor. In 1971 a dormitory with a capacity of twelve students was added to again offer residential treatment to those youngsters needing the most intensive care. And in 1986, to accommodate youths who had aged out of the Linwood programs, Linwood opened its first group home for adults.

JEANNE'S METHODS WERE empirically derived, based on her training and her understanding, underpinned by her personal experiences of the challenges children living with autism face. Her approach required patience and an extended period of close, careful observation before interventions were attempted. During an initial intake period the child was pretty much left to his own devices; this helped identify his unique behavior patterns and strengths, which could then be used to gradually help him move toward more productive behaviors.

Since these children have difficulties with change, it was seen as important to give them time to become familiar with a specific setting that always included one or more of the same adults. This welcoming and initially unchanging environment and the therapists' acceptance of each child and his behaviors created an atmosphere of safety that allowed children to venture out of old, "safe"—although dysfunctional—patterns. Jeanne called this "establishing a relationship," but what it amounts to is not the kind of personal bond we imagine when we talk about "relationships," but the establishment of familiarity and basic trust between the child and the teacher.

Rather than working on suppressing symptoms that might interfere with learning or following a pre-set schedule, the focus at Linwood was always on identifying areas of health that could be worked with. It was the child who set the pace, and his needs determined the priorities.

Importantly, the Linwood staff looked for "natural" rewards, things derived from each individual child's own needs, interests, or preoccupations. External rewards such as tokens, toys, or food, though given brief trials, were seen as less lastingly effective than letting the child experience the consequences of his own actions; natural rewards acted as both motivators and inhibitors, gradually producing new, more adaptive behaviors. Praise or explicit approval were at most used as reinforcers with children who had already made significant progress toward normal functioning, since most children with autism spectrum disorder (ASD) do not care about another's reactions and feelings. It was also understood that progress was rarely linear, and a period of progress was frequently followed by one of regression.

Children were assigned to classrooms according to their level of functioning. As they progressed, increasingly formal school content was added to their routine, but the sequence of the acquisition of discrete skills always followed the child's lead.

THE 1975 Education for All Handicapped Children Act (PL94-142) significantly changed the educational environment, though for a long time teachers in public and most private schools did not know what to make of children with ASD or how to provide them with an adequate learning experience. As interest in autism spectrum disorder grew, autism research began to find its way into medical books and professional journals. And as public funding became more available, centers dedicated to the study and treatment of the condition started to proliferate.

While the Linwood method had revolutionized the early treatment and education of children with ASD, it began to become overshadowed by and eventually subsumed into more formalized approaches collectively known as *applied behavioral analysis* (ABA). These methods were all based on B. F. Skinner's early experiments with the operant conditioning of animals.

Prominent among the professionals studying and working with models based on operant conditioning was the clinical psychologist Ole Ivar Lovaas. In the 1950s he became known for helping to pioneer a method of behavior modification that used excessively adverse interventions (electroshock) to extinguish severe self-aggressive behaviors in children with autism and other severe disabilities. Jeanne knew of his work and along with the whole autism community abhorred and condemned it. But because of his later work, in the 1970s and 1980s, at the Neuropsychiatric Institute of UCLA, where he started an early intervention clinic, he became identified as "the father of ABA" and its offspring, evidence-based teaching, especially discrete trial training (DTT). Since the late 1990s these methods have been the gold standard for teaching and therapy with autistic children. A number of colleges and universities teach them and certify teachers to use them with children who have ASD.

Lovaas is also commonly credited with having been the first to provide evidence that the behavior of children with autism could be modified through teaching, even though such evidence was demonstrated daily at Linwood long before his ascendance.

One of the reasons operant conditioning methods embodied by ABA became better known than the approach pioneered by Jeanne was that Linwood was a private institution, unaffiliated with a university or research center. And, while Lovaas and his colleagues published hundreds of research articles and a number of books in the 1970s and 1980s, Jeanne had not systematically analyzed her approach or written it down until *The Hidden Child*, which was not published until 1987 (1). Jeanne's methods seeded centers worldwide through interns, visiting professionals, and some collaborative work with colleagues in other countries. But she taught by example. There was little research coming out of Linwood, with only two research papers ever published to alert the professional world to the work being done there.

One was an article by the behavioral psychologist Charles B. Ferster, an adherent of Skinner and a pioneer in behavior modification whose work Jeanne mentions in chapter 12. With a research grant from the US Department of Health, Education, and Welfare for a three-year study beginning in 1966 of the methods used at Linwood, Ferster's intent was to demonstrate that principles of behavioral conditioning used with animals could be taught to the staff to make them more effective therapists with developmentally disabled children. To his and the staff's surprise it turned out that the approach developed by Jeanne, while at first glance nothing like the operant conditioning methods made famous by Skinner and his disciples, was already using principles of behavioral conditioning without ever identifying them as such. Before Ferster's analysis, the often dramatic improvements of children placed at Linwood were regarded as sheer magic by some dazzled observers; it took Ferster to identify the discrete behavior modification components in the work done there and how they were incorporated into a total treatment approach.

The only published piece to come out of Ferster's research, an early account of his observations, was an article written and published with Jeanne in 1966 (2). Unfortunately, he never published his observations and insights once his three-year study was completed. A paper titled "An Operant Analysis of Infantile Autism," which he wrote as he wrapped up his work, remained unpublished. Educational and academic institutions and the autism community therefore remained ignorant that a hugely successful method of behavior modification developed by a uniquely gifted teacher was practiced and thriving at Linwood decades before such methods were formalized and enshrined in ABA.

Concurrent with Ferster's research, Dr. Kanner examined thirty-four children at Linwood in 1966. He discovered that while all of them were dysfunctional, they had varying diagnoses. Of the group he identified fifteen with autism (thirteen boys and two girls). He reevaluated all these youngsters in1968 and those then still at Linwood again in 1973, with Jeanne assisting in their follow-up evaluations. He published his findings in 1973 together with notes by Jeanne about each child's development up to the date of publication (3).

Although Kanner noted that further research would be needed to meaningfully relate the outcome to diagnosis and duration of time at Linwood, Jeanne's approach had led to significant improvements in the functioning of fourteen of the fifteen children with autism. By 1973 eight had moved on from Linwood to special day care centers; another six had "attained a state of near full or full recovery," in the sense that they had transitioned to regular public schools and were living at home. Only one ended up in an institution. And only a few of the original cohort tested "had demonstrated no visible progress."

But the Linwood method, though clearly successful when looked at over time, did not lend itself to the kind of accountability that public funders demanded. While Linwood students of school age all had an individualized educational plan (IEP), the program did not follow a published guide with pre-set goals that could be charted day to day and statistically quantified, like teaching guides built into all ABA-based programs. And by the 1990s, the physical plant no longer satisfied modern requirements. It lacked flexible spaces, modern teaching aides and equipment, lab space, and other amenities deemed essential for an up-to-date school.

Other, better-equipped, centers that had adopted the ABA approach had opened in the Baltimore-Washington area and nationwide and were turning out a slew of research documentation of their successes, while Linwood went about its business out of the public eye. Additionally, requirements for community-based treatment moved treatment away from residential treatment facilities to community settings, so the dormitory had to be closed and community housing provided for those young people who could not be maintained at home.

From a thriving community in the late 1980s, Linwood's descent toward obscurity and insolvency was shockingly fast. Referring school systems lost confidence in Linwood. It was losing hundreds of thousands of dollars every year, and by 2005, the year Jeanne died and Linwood celebrated its fiftieth anniversary, the center was barely on life support.

What happened next is vividly described by Bill Moss, who had come to Linwood as an intern in 1975 and together with a couple of other promising young teachers had been groomed by Jeanne to take over from her once she retired. He was the only one left of this trium-virate to help prevent Linwood from having to close down. (He re-tired in September of 2019 after forty-five years of service to Lin-wood.) This is how Moss described what happened in the late 1990s and into the new century:

> Linwood was on the verge of extinction. To save it, we made some tough decisions that cost us the leadership as it existed during the last decades of the Simons years (with one exception—me). The very first thing I did when I was appointed as executive director in 2002 was to put on a coat and tie and attend as many meetings in as many arenas as I could. I was rarely in the office. Just by doing that, enrollment increased from twenty-four students to thirty students. We brought on a community outreach director for a couple of years. Between us, we identified exactly what our stakeholders wanted that we were not giving them.
>
> Based on that information, we developed a five-year strategic plan and began a capital campaign to build a new school. Between the state, the county, and privately raised funds, we raised half the money we needed and borrowed the other half. We also rein-vented our programs. We hired a very young staff and put them in charge. They came in with new ideas, a new focused approach, while there were still a few of us old-timers helping to steer the ship so we didn't veer too far off course. Enrollment exploded and the center became self-sustaining. It is actually what Jeanne Simons did in her day, except on a much grander scale.

Moss also insisted that despite the change in name and additional bells and whistles, the basic spirit of the treatment and the treatment principles established by Jeanne were alive and well at Linwood and were incorporated not only into its practices but into the treatment approaches of most reputable institutions.

One of the better-known such programs is the Early Start Denver Model. It uses a developmentally based, child-led curriculum for children ages twelve to forty-eight months. A range of other programs, such as pivotal response treatment, or PRT, are integrated into a child's own environment and emphasize natural reinforcers. Most such programs emphasize parent training so that a consistent environment can be maintained for a child—a difference from Linwood, where parents were advised and supported but were not expected to formally work with their children.

THE NEW LINWOOD CENTER operates in an educational environment that is vastly different from the one in place in 1955 and the following three decades. In good part changes came about through a growing awareness that developmentally impaired children needed levels of care that at the time were not available in the public school system—and were available in only a few private institutions and at a cost that was beyond the means of most affected families. With the influx of public monies, programs in both the public and the nonpublic sectors proliferated in the late 1980s, with levels of care for every condition and need.

Insights gained about the neurological development of young brains also suggested that early interventions with developmentally disabled children, including those diagnosed with ASD, was crucial for more positive later outcomes. Every county in Maryland now has some type of early intervention program, mostly delivered in the home. They all come with formal educational objectives and the goal to get children ready for some type of primary school program.

Because more public schools now have programs for children with various disabilities, an early selection process will already have taken place by the time a child applies to Linwood. Higher-functioning children and those whose behaviors do not majorly interfere with their ability to learn are being triaged into public schools. Consequently, around 80% of the present school-age population at Linwood are moderately to severely intellectually impaired and on average function at a first- or second-grade level. The center offers an academic curriculum that runs through middle school for the other children, but it does not presently have a regular high school program, so older children who are on track for a high school diploma have to be transferred to centers that do. Linwood also cannot accommodate children with severe physical handicaps, significant medical needs, or comorbidity that is so severe that such disabilities would require interventions beyond the available parameters.

All children who enter Linwood—at the earliest at age five—already come with documentation of their level of functioning and an initial individualized educational plan. It is the referring public school that sets the educational standards for each child and together with the parents and the Linwood staff develops subsequent IEPs each year. Linwood has to provide the schools with regular progress reports including data on the measurable criteria that were set for each goal in the IEP. While the center is a nongraded school with children roughly grouped by age, all students pursue their own individual academic and behavioral goals. The ultimate goal for every child is to be placed in a public school setting, though, as the children age, vocational skills training takes on greater importance.

Children generally enter Linwood with behaviors that interfere not only with their ability to learn but also with their social functioning. The former is relevant to their ability to acquire academic skills, the latter to their functioning within a classroom or group setting and ultimately to their ability to transition into an adult program. So, while attempting to impart basic academic skills and track and document academic progress, the teachers also have to help each child to learn to modify dysfunctional and disruptive behaviors and replace them with more functional ones. And this progress, too, has to be tracked and documented. Having to address all of these challenges more or less simultaneously requires not only highly trained special education teachers with additional certification in working with children with ASD, but individuals with a keen sense of observation, infinite patience, and the ability to stay calm and organized under stress—a combination that is rare and precious.

Linwood also has a large nonverbal population requiring various specialized approaches. The center employs a full-time speech and language specialist who develops individualized strategies to foster communications and verbal skills. To develop early communications skills Linwood uses a tool also used in early intervention programs for younger children, the VB-MAPP (Verbal Behavior Milestone Assessment and Placement Program). It is both a curriculum guide and a system to track developing communications skills.

Nonverbal children are taught a variety of communication modes, often in combination, that can include signing as well as typed communication on a computer or picture communication. Early verbal skills are enabled by a system called augmentative alternative communication, or ACC. Each child receives a tablet that can be individualized with pictures and matching vocabulary words he may be working on. The tablet may have a symbol that when tapped calls up pictures of various emotions, so he can indicate his state of mind, and another symbol for preferred foods or activities, or for family members, among many other options. On the one hand the tablet provides a means of communication that might eventually lead to verbal speech; on the other it is a way to associate word prompts with pictures and a written word, enlarging the vocabulary. The ultimate goal is to generalize concepts, so that the word *cat*, for example, prompts the child not only to choose the correct picture but to identify a live cat.

To move children forward toward competency in set areas, the school uses the basic tools of operant conditioning as outlined in discrete trial training. When teaching new tasks with this method, prompts are initially given but are then faded out as the behavior is exhibited more reliably. For early learners, motivators to move toward a desired goal are food or the use of a favorite toy or activity, given immediately after the task has been done.

In one classroom I observed a student who was clearly uninterested in completing the task of answering a question by choosing between two pictures. He was given several prompts by the teaching assistant slightly waving the correct picture. The picture then had to be glued onto a sheet of paper. Again, the child showed no interest in completing the task. The adult briefly let him see a small bag of cookies she had in her pocket, which was enough to get him to stick on a couple more pictures, thus earning him the morsel of cookie. Once the whole group had completed the task they had a free period during which each child claimed his own space and activity in a playroom, seemingly unaware of the presence of other children, staff, or the observer in the room.

Children who have made more progress are switched from food or other immediate rewards to what could be called a "token economy." A successfully executed task is rewarded with some kind of token that can later be used to "buy" a reward, with an ascending number of tokens needed to get the reward, be it iPod use, time on the playground, or some other activity the child enjoys.

Techniques for modifying or extinguishing dysfunctional behaviors depend on the severity of the behavior as well as their meaning to the child. For severely dysfunctional behaviors, the goal is extinction; for less severe ones, either moderation or replacement behaviors that augment a child's ability to function socially.

Modifiers are geared to both the severity of the undesirable behavior and the level of functioning of a child. For more advanced children, for example, the removal of a token alone may be effective. If the behavior's purpose is to seek attention, ignoring it is the preferred tactic. This is also the case with behaviors a child engages in to avoid or escape a task. In that case, focusing on the disruptive behavior reinforces that behavior, since it was obviously successful and acts as "negative reinforcement." "Escape extinction" avoids that pitfall by continuing to focus on the task at hand, ignoring the avoidance behaviors as much as possible.

The modeling of replacement behaviors, paired with positive redirection, is another technique that has proven successful. If a child is extremely agitated or dangerously aggressive, a brief isolation in a "quiet room" may be effective, with a staff member present right outside the door to gauge the child's readiness to rejoin his group.

The school's staff is keenly aware of the need to prepare the children in their care for the transition into adult life in the least restrictive environment possible. A youngster with better self-help and social skills has a much better chance to be accepted into supported adult programs, housing, and employment. This is important not only because such programs promise a better quality of life, but because financial support after age twenty-one becomes much harder to access and the long-term outlook for those not accepted into a supported program is less positive. The autism waiver program, for example, only applies to individuals under age twenty-one.

SINCE THE YEAR 2000, Linwood's budget has grown from $2.8 to $14 million. It now has a staff of two hundred and fifty employees. Funding comes from a number of sources, but central to all of the funding are the ideas that people with developmental disabilities need to be placed in the least restrictive environment and that all of their care needs to be community based.

For its present population of fifty-three children, ages five to twenty-one, Linwood employs eleven teachers and four behavior specialists as well as a music therapist, instructional assistants, and a transition coordinator, among others, as well as a nurse dedicated to the school population (though clients use outside psychiatrists for needed psychotropic medications). Social workers and a dedicated behavioral team design wrap-around services in partnership with the families to assure consistent care and seamless transitions. Linwood also works with the neurobehavioral unit at the Kennedy Krieger Institute in Baltimore and refers children in crisis to Sheppard Pratt in Towson, Maryland.

Most of the children live at home, though eleven youngsters between the ages of twelve and twenty-one are residentially placed in apartments throughout the community, either because of problems in the home or because of transportation issues that would interfere with school attendance. Most of them live in groups of three to four per home, with an equal number of staff, which makes their care very expensive.

It is Linwood's adult population that has grown the fastest, standing at seventy-five as of this account. Linwood's growth in adult population reflects the national trend that predicts that over the next ten years an additional fifty thousand adults with the autism spectrum diagnosis per year will need services in the United States alone. Linwood serves its adult patients according to their specific needs through a number of therapeutic and supportive programs, all of them community based: Forty adults live in community housing, mostly owned and wholly staffed by Linwood. All of them either are in day habilitation programs to acquire prerequisite work skills or work in facilities that accommodate supported employment (paid for by Medicare and Medicaid), in which co-workers and supervisors are trained to deal with the adult's particular needs. They can also be shadowed on the job, if necessary. Personal support in the home can also be delivered by Linwood staff, though funding for such services is limited.

THE LINWOOD CENTER OF TODAY is no longer the Linwood of Jeanne Simons, but when she retired, she not only was prepared to see it change under new leadership but believed that such change was a natural and necessary process, and that Linwood would be "evolving like any living organism." What was important to her above all else was that those who because of their vulnerabilities could not be accommodated at home or in a regular educational environment should not be lost, given up on, or "warehoused." Linwood today valiantly fulfills that legacy.

REFERENCES

1. Simons, J., & Oishi, S. The Hidden Child: The Linwood Method for Reaching the Autistic Child. Baltimore, MD: Woodbine House, 1987.
2. Ferster, C. B., & Simons, J. Behavior therapy with children. Psychological Record 1966; 16:65–71.
3. Kanner, L. Childhood Psychosis: Initial Studies and New Insights. New York: John Wiley and Sons, 1973.

Afterword

James C. Harris, MD

Both Jeanne Simons and Leo Kanner were tireless advocates for individualized treatment for children with autism spectrum disorders, recognizing the children as unique persons, and were selflessly devoted to their care. Jeanne, as a teacher, exhibited a remarkable ethical concern in her advocacy for children that is vividly described in this book. Working at a Catholic institution in the Netherlands for deprived youth who were harshly treated and poorly fed, she confronted the institution's board members by serving them the same gruel served to the children. That got their attention! Her advocacy led to substantial changes in child care at the institution with the provision of new warm clothing and decent meals. The story of her escape from war-torn Europe in the 1940s rescuing a young child in her care to the safety in the United States is harrowing.

Psychiatrist Leo Kanner's advocacy for children with developmental disorders began in the 1930s. In 1942, the year before his autism paper was published, Kanner debated neurologist Foster Kennedy of Columbia University in the *American Journal of Psychiatry* about whether children with severe intellectual disability should be euthanized in the United States, as they were being in Nazi Germany, as "life unworthy of life" (1). The neurologist proposed that, with parental permission, euthanasia (killing such children) was permissible (2). Kanner adamantly insisted that such killing is unethical. He titled his paper "Exoneration of the [Intellectually Disabled]."

I was inspired by Jeanne Simons and Leo Kanner's advocacy throughout my residency training in psychiatry. My experience treating a child with autism began with John, the child who stimulated my interest in his treatment. He was a bright boy who avoided eye contact. Our sessions commenced using a typewriter, taking turns typing messages back and forth to each other. One day, after several months working together, he typed that Alison, his sister, was crying. I typed "Alison is sad." He alerted, looked directly at me, and excitedly said, "Oh, Yes." That was beginning of his recognition of emotion, that is, recognizing the feeling of sadness in his sister. Jeanne had told me a similar story about emotion realization in a boy she treated at Linwood. One day he came to her and reminded her that several years before, when he was seated at a table with other boys, he suddenly knocked over the table and ran out of the room. In a moment of emotional awareness he told Jeanne that that day she had paid more attention to another boy than to him, and he had rebelled. In this moment of emotional recognition, he shouted to her that it was "jealousy."

Jeanne's life story is remarkable in revealing that as an adult she realized she was on the autism spectrum. Her siblings, when they visited Linwood, confirmed the similarity between the autistic behavior of the children treated there with her behavior as a child. Seeking the origins of her autistic features, Jeanne attributes birth hypoxia, a recognized environmental risk factor for autism spectrum disorder, as the cause (3). Family support and self-determination may account for Jeanne's ability to cope with and master her autistic symptoms. She writes, "I am convinced that my autism is not innate but is the result of birth trauma, especially oxygen deprivation. Therefore, I think that I had the potential to relate normally. It was only through an accident of birth that I became so abnormally sensitive to the emotions engendered by human interactions that I couldn't tolerate them and had to close off from them. I had to protect myself against them or be destroyed."

During Jeanne's long lifetime (1909–2005) and afterward, significant advances have been made in the diagnosis, classification, and treatment of autism. These developments are described in appendix A. Moreover, appendix A discusses reasons why the numbers of people diagnosed with autism have increased, and reviews genetic and environmental causes of autism. It summarizes the importance of, and the application of, advances in developmental social and cognitive neuroscience in early case identification, in finding biomarkers, and mapping brain circuits that will inform future diagnosis and treatments.

In conclusion, I am grateful for the pioneering work of Jeanne Simons, Leo Kanner, and the multitude of their successors that has made possible the remarkable advances being made in improving the lives of children with autism spectrum disorder diagnoses and their families.

REFERENCES

1. Kanner, L. Exoneration of the feebleminded [intellectually disabled]. American Journal of Psychiatry 1942; 99:17–22.
2. Kennedy, F. The problem of social control of the congenital defective: education, sterilization, euthanasia. American Journal of Psychiatry 1942; 99:13–16.
3. Modabbernia, A., Velthorst, E., & Reichenberg, A. Environmental risk factors for autism: An evidence-based review of systematic reviews and meta-analyses. Molecular Autism 2017; 8(1):13.

Appendix A
A brief overview of autism spectrum disorder
Diagnostic criteria, research, and treatment
James C. Harris, MD

The evolving diagnosis and classification of autism

In 1908 Eugen Bleuler (1857–1939), a leading Swiss professor of psychiatry, introduced the term *autism* (withdrawal from reality) as a symptom of schizophrenia (1). In the 1940s Leo Kanner (1894–1981) credited Bleuler when he proposed the term *early infantile autism* in a different context than Bleuler to describe young children with a neurodevelopmental disorder. Kanner wrote that "these children have come into the world with an innate inability to form the usual, biologically provided contact with people" and to socially engage with others, just as other children are born with innate physical problems like cerebral palsy (2). He emphasized their autistic aloneness, resistance to change, echolalia, increased sensitivity to sound or other sensory stimulation, and stereotypical repetitive behaviors (such as hand flapping and spinning), and recognized their exceptionally good memory. Moreover, Kanner's recognition of autistic traits in many of their parents set the stage for later recognition of the importance of genetic factors in autism and the identification of the broader autism phenotype in families.

In the first and second editions of the American Psychiatric Association's *Diagnostic and Statistical Manual of Mental Disorders*, autism was classified as *infantile psychosis* (loss of contact with reality), and *early infantile autism* was not clearly recognized as diagnostically different from *early onset schizophrenia*. With publication of the third edition of the manual, *DSM-III*, in 1980, autism was defined as a *pervasive developmental disorder* that involved disturbed development in social understanding, language use, attention, and perception, formalizing Kanner's original description (3). The most striking symptoms of the disorder were listed as an absence of social self-awareness in relationship to others and lack of the use of the imagination in adapting to everyday life. Infants with this disorder fail to initiate personal contact by reaching to be picked up, ignore people in their surroundings, and seem to be in a "world of their own."

An "autistic savant's" special numerical calculation abilities were depicted by Dustin Hoffman in the movie *Rain Man*. The movie's director arranged for Hoffman to meet young men diagnosed with autism (one of them was from Linwood) to learn to mimic autistic behaviors. Savant skills are rare in people with autism, however. When they do occur, they are most often the result of constant practice and extreme preoccupation with a particular subject. However, as we have seen with Jeanne Simons' Lee, who was able to attribute dates and days of the weeks over decades, savant skills are not unknown.

More common traits across the autism spectrum are "literalness," which together with a lack of imagination typically results in an inability to lie or dissemble; repetitive motor movements and rituals; and extreme distress at small changes in routine or environment. For example, the insistence on the same food, same routes, and same routines; and difficulties with transitions. A striking symptom is an apparent indifference to pain. Also frequently encountered are extreme sensitivity to sensory stimuli, sometimes expressed in excessive smelling and touching of objects and fascination with lights or movement or negative reactions to certain sounds. In 2013, excessive sensitivity was included as a criterion in *DSM-5*.

In the 1980 edition of the *Diagnostic and Statistical Manual of Mental Disorders* (*DSM-III*), specific criteria for early infantile autism were introduced. These criteria were broadened in a 1987 revision of the manual (*DSM-III-R*), and the name was changed *from early infantile autism* to *autistic disorder* (4). The earlier criteria were viewed as too limited in focusing on infants and too restrictive by only focusing on more severely involved children. Thus, revised criteria were needed to facilitate diagnosis in childhood and to include milder cases. However, when implemented, these new, revised criteria were found to be too broad, leading to too many false positive cases, resulting in a further text revision, in *DSM-IV* in 1994 (5).

Moreover, *DSM-IV* established *subtypes* of pervasive developmental disorder. The best known among them was *Asperger's syndrome*, originally *autistic psychopathy*, first proposed in 1944 by the Austrian pediatrician Hans Asperger (1906–1980), the year after Kanner's paper was published. Asperger described *autistic psychopathy* (6); the name later changed to *Asperger syndrome* (7), as a personality disorder typically recognized in childhood rather than in infancy. The children he described had difficulty in understanding social relationships, atypical language development, and perseverative interests. They differed from Kannner's cases in age of first recognition, in having better language ability, and, over all, higher cognitive functioning. Importantly, Asperger and Kanner always viewed the syndromes they described as distinct. However, when the diagnostic criteria for Asperger's syndrome in *DSM-IV* were examined in larger samples of children, research findings concluded that Asperger's syndrome could not be clearly differentiated from high-functioning autism. This led to the elimination of Asperger syndrome as a category in *DSM-5* (8).

In fact, the current *Diagnostic Manual, DSM-5*, eliminates all of the *DSM-IV* subtypes in favor of a new general category, *autism spectrum disorder (ASD)* (8). Kanner's syndrome (early infantile autism) and Asperger's syndrome (autistic psychopathy) are both now classified as autism spectrum disorders. The term *spectrum* refers to a variety of autistic presentations and not to the severity of the presentation. Severity is further classified by the extent of needed supports in social communication and with restricted and repetitive behaviors as Level 1 (requiring support), Level 2 (requiring substantial support), and Level 3 (requiring very substantial support). Moreover, in *DSM-5* the number of defining criteria are reduced from three criteria domains (social behavior, communication deficits, and restrictive and repetitive behaviors) into two criteria domains (impaired social communication / interactions and restrictive and repetitive behaviors). The change was made to clarify that communication refers specifically to social communication. Hyper- or hyporeactivity to sensory input or unusual interest in sensory aspects of the environment was added as a new criterion. Autism spectrum disorder can be present with or without accompanying intellectual impairment and with or without language impairment and may be associated with several neurogenetic syndromes (9, 10).

Significantly, a new category, *social communication disorder* (SCD), is introduced in *DSM-5* under the section on communication disorders (8). This is a disorder of pragmatic language, that is, in the social use of language, without the repetitive behavior features seen in typical autism. This new category accounts for some pervasive developmental disorders–not otherwise specified (PDD-NOS) cases and addresses a problem in *DSM-IV* of co-occurrence of autism with other diagnoses like attention-deficit/hyperactivity disorder (ADHD). It is of interest historically that one of Leo Kanner's colleagues in child psychiatry at Johns Hopkins, Georg Frankl, published an accompanying article in the same issue of the journal *The Nervous Child* where Kanner's autism article appeared in 1943. Frankl's article was titled "Language and Affective Contact" (11). Frankl described a child with tuberous sclerosis who had deficits in pragmatic language; today, using *DSM-5* criteria, this child would be diagnosed with a *social communication disorder.*

DSM-5 is documented as an improvement over *DSM-IV* in the early recognition of cases.

The increasing prevalence of autism spectrum disorder

The introduction of *DSM-5* has not been shown to meaningfully change the prevalence of the disorder, though with the broadening of the diagnostic criteria in the various revisions of the *DSM* the number of cases identified has dramatically increased. In Leo Kanner's time through the 1970s, before *DSM-III* was introduced, autism was estimated as occurring in fewer than 1 per 1,000 in the general population. In 2000, the Centers for Disease Control and Prevention (CDC) Autism and Developmental Disability Monitoring (ADDM) Network began regularly reporting on the prevalence of autism spectrum disorder using *DSM-IV* criteria in eight-year-old children at thirteen sites around the country. The prevalence was estimated as 6.7 per 1,000, or 1 in 150. In 2014 the estimate was 16.8 per 1,000: 1 in 59 children, or 1.7% of the population, have the diagnosis (12). Comparing *DSM-IV* criteria and *DSM-5* criteria, the CDC reports that ASD prevalence was approximately 4% higher using the *DSM-IV* criteria. Comparing *DSM-IV* and *DSM-5* criteria in a subset of four-year-old children at three of the thirteen sites used for the study of eight-year-olds, the prevalence reported in this age group was 20% higher with *DSM-IV* than with the *DSM-5* criteria (17.0 per 1,000 versus 14.1 per 1,000, respectively) (13). However, overall the prevalence in four-year-olds was unchanged in two of the three sites and higher in one. Overall increases in prevalence over time suggest a near epidemic, but much of the increase is believed to be due to more inclusive and detailed diagnostic criteria that include higher-functioning children.

Another factor that may contribute to the higher prevalence is the far greater attention being paid to making the diagnosis after the federal government mandated that special education services be provided for children with ASD. In 1990, the US government, with Public Law Number 101-476, added autism as a new special education disability category in amendments to PL 94-142, the Education for All Handicapped Children Act (14). Now called the Disabilities Education Act, this law requires funding for early identification and intervention. Once the school system was required to provide special educational services for children with ASD, parents increasingly pressured pediatricians and psychiatrists to make the diagnosis so their child could obtain services, a factor that has influenced greater recognition and inclusion of milder presentations.

Autism spectrum disorder occurs in all racial and socioeconomic groups but, overall, boys are approximately four times more likely to be diagnosed than girls. Using current criteria, studies in North America, Europe, and Asia find a 1% to 2% population prevalence, so the increase in recognition is not limited to the United States. The United Nations Convention on Rights of Persons with Disabilities calls for necessary accommodations and supports for people with an autism diagnosis (15).

Kanner recognized diagnostic heterogeneity and opined that the children "had not read" the diagnostic manuals and did not easily fall into clear-cut categories (16, p. 347). The current high rates may bear out Kanner's concerns in the 1960s, when he wrote that it had "become a habit to dilute the original concept of autism by diagnosing it in many disparate conditions which show one or another isolated feature found as a part feature of the overall syndrome." He suggested that the country seemed to be becoming overpopulated with a multitude of children with autism. The high prevalence suggests that current criteria may be too broad. Future classifications may be based on new research identifying new and better defined subtypes so treatment can be better targeted (17). In keeping with Kanner's concern about diluting the original concept of autism, there is growing concern today that too often the diagnosis is made based on autism screening checklists that lack diagnostic specificity. These rating scales are meant to be screening instruments only, and are to be followed up with referrals for comprehensive assessment. Those assessments typically include the Autism Diagnostic Interview (ADI) and the Autism Diagnostic Observation Schedule (ADOS).

Always an advocate for children, Kanner, when reviewing the *DSM-III* criteria in 1980, emphasized that no matter how well developed our criteria, each child must be treated as a unique person. At Linwood, Jeanne Simons worked with the most severely involved cases recognized by Kanner and others in the 1950s and later. It is this population who continue to be those in most need of services. The parent advocacy group the National Autism Association strongly advocates for such services. Jeanne led the way in treating each child as unique person and focused less on diagnostic criteria and more on focusing on each child's uniqueness.

What causes autism?

No single gene, but many genes, have been found that may contribute to autism. Identification of these genes, as described below, has led to the testing of clusters of genes that may increase risk. These clusters are referred to as *polygenic risk scores* (18). At the time Kanner described autism, the field of genetics was in its infancy and medical research showed little interest in inborn psychiatric disorders. The anti-genetic zeitgeist ascendant in those years emphasized that what mattered most were environmental factors, especially parental neglect and harsh responses to their children's behavior. Little was known about treatment, and these children were commonly institutionalized.

Yet, Leo Kanner rejected parental neglect as a cause of autism. Kanner often used metaphors in his teaching. In his introductory lecture to child psychiatrists, Kanner said that if children were overly protected (by what today are called helicopter parents) it was like being raised in an emotional oven, and if rejected it was like being raised in an emotional refrigerator. It is a major misunderstanding to claim that Kanner blamed parents. He did recognize autistic traits in many of the children's parents, but he did not blame them for causing their children's condition; he simply described their behavior. He found they did not reject their children; nor did they abuse them. These parents sought his help. He was very supportive of mothers and in 1941 published a book, *In Defense of Mothers*, to encourage them to follow their natural instincts in child-rearing (19). In the 1960s, Kanner expressed concern about psychiatrists and psychologists blaming mothers for causing autism when he wrote, "There was a tendency in this country to view [autism] as a developmental anomaly ascribed exclusively to maternal emotional determinants" (20, p. 413).

However, others insisted that parental behavior was the cause. In 1948 Frieda Fromm-Reichman proposed the term *schizophrenogenic mother* as a cause for schizophrenia, a view that persisted into the 1950s and 1960s until it was finally abandoned (21). It was Bruno Bettelheim (1903–1990), who became director of the Orthogenic School in Chicago in 1944, who popularized the term *refrigerator mother* as the cause of autism. He is worthy of note because he was very influential in treating disturbed children, many with autistic-like behaviors, though he had no formal training or background in psychology or psychiatry. Bettelheim was an Austrian Jew and self-styled psychoanalyst who survived a brief incarceration in two concentration camps. He likened the children's behavior to that of concentration camp victims who had given up hope and become totally passive, then ascribed their behavior to mothers—who, he said, must have treated their children like cruel and persecuting camp guards. In his 1967 book *The Empty Fortress,* Bettelheim speculated that refrigerator mothers who were unresponsive to their children predisposed them to autism. He wrote that "the precipitating factor in infantile autism is the parent's wish that [their] child did not exist" (22, p. 125).

Kanner was appalled at Bettelheim's views. As the guest of honor at the first meeting of the National Society for Autistic Children (NSAC; now named the Autism Society of America), he made clear he had never blamed parents and, in typical good humor, said he exonerated them all. Kanner told the audience: "From the very first publication until the last, I spoke of this condition in no uncertain terms as 'innate.' But because I described some of the characteristics of the parents as persons, I was mis-quoted often as having said that 'it is all the parents' fault.' Those of you parents who have come to see me with your children know that this isn't what I said. As a matter of fact, I have tried to relieve parental anxiety when they had been made anxious because of such speculation" (23, p. 226). Kanner received a standing ovation and was given a plaque by NSAC to commemorate his contributions.

Although Kanner clearly stated that the parents did not cause autism, he did not say that the environment did not matter. He noted that the "emotional configuration of the home does play a dynamic role" in the child's ongoing development. Child-rearing practices do matter. Understanding this, Kanner was delighted when Jeanne Simons developed an approach in which interventions focused on providing positive emotional support targeted the needs of each child. Indeed, Jeanne's decision to open Linwood was driven in good part by her empathy with the parents of children who were too difficult to maintain safely in a home environment.

Genetic factors

In the years following Kanner's first publication, research has convincingly demonstrated the importance of genetics in understanding autism. Kanner's early recognition of parental personal traits—specifically, that parents he evaluated typically were overly focused on details and showed limited interest in social interactions—set the stage for the later identification of genetic factors associated with the *broader autism phenotype*. The broader autism phenotype refers to the presence of mild ASD symptoms in a family that do not meet strict diagnostic criteria for ASD.

Genetic studies in identical twins confirmed a genetic basis of autism (24). A review of more than thirteen twin studies found that 45% of identical twins had the diagnosis of autism compared to 15% of nonidentical (fraternal) twins (25, p. 103). Genetic studies examine rearrangements of chromosomes in children with an autism diagnosis to identify genetic mutations (25, p. 103; 26). Despite advances in genetics, however, approximately 90% of cases have not been found to have a known genetic disorder syndrome. About 10% of people diagnosed, primarily those who also have an intellectual developmental disorder, have inherited a genetic syndrome or have a new mutation.

Because autism spectrum disorder risk is influenced by both commonly known genes and rare new mutations, efforts are underway to establish co-occurrence of multiple-risk genes. Combining multiple-risk genes, as noted above, is referred to as a *polygenic risk score*. This method is being used to study subgroups of ASD cases. Using this method, a polygenic genetic transmission disequilibrium test was carried out in 6,454 families to calculate polygenic risk for ASD separate from IQ test score. Polygenic variation was found to contribute to risk in ASD cases who had rare severe new mutation ASD risk variants (27). Next steps are underway to identify distinct causative pathways.

Environmental factors

Compared to genetic studies of autism spectrum disorder, there are far fewer studies of environmental risk factors such as birth anoxia. However, Jeanne was correct in proposing her autism was linked to hypoxia. Birth hypoxia and birth complications have strong links to ASD (28). Hypoxic-ischemic birth effects on the brain include inflammation, oxidative damage, and excitotoxicity that may act independently or interact with family genetic background leading to an ASD diagnosis. Lack of oxygen alters brain cell energy metabolism and may lead to brain cell dysfunction and death of cells. Brain regions involved in cognition—that is, in acquiring knowledge and understanding through thought, experience, and the senses—are commonly injured following lack of oxygen at birth (neonatal hypoxia). Such regions primarily involve the hippocampus, which is involved in the consolidation of information from short-term memory to long-term memory and in spatial memory, and the cerebral cortex, which is involved in thinking, perceiving, producing, and understanding language.

One study provides insight into possible mechanisms of hypoxic damage to the brain that is pertinent to ASD. This study found that lack of oxygen at birth affects brain proteins that are involved in two known genetic syndromes with autistic features, Fragile X syndrome and tuberous sclerosis complex (29). For example, the Fragile X protein plays an important role in the development of brain neurons, dendritic spine development, and the function of brain synapses. When brain tissues of newborns with hypoxic-ischemic brain damage were compared to healthy controls in this study, significantly lower Fragile X protein amounts were found in the hippocampus and cortical brain regions of those with hypoxic damage than in those without it (29). This study proposes that disruption of the Fragile X protein and the tuberous sclerosis protein pathways may be a mechanism where hypoxic-ischemic damage could be linked to ASD.

Advances in treatments for autism spectrum disorders

Beginning in 1955, Jean Simons began working closely with Leo Kanner to provide an optimal treatment environment for children with autism at Linwood. Her approach is described in *The Hidden Child* (30). As she describes in chapter 12, she collaborated with Charles B. Ferster, a leading operant behavioral psychologist who had studied with B. F. Skinner and later became the head of the department of psychology at American University in Washington, DC. Dr. Kanner examined thirty-four children from Linwood with varying diagnoses beginning in 1966. He did follow-ups in 1968 and again in 1973 and published his findings (31).

Substantial refinements have been made in the treatment of autism since Kanner's report of successful treatment at Linwood nearly fifty years ago. Elements of the Linwood approach are now incorporated into school programs nationally. The Linwood program demonstrated that children with an autism spectrum disorder respond to warm, empathic-focused psychosocial treatments.

Once children are diagnosed with an autism spectrum disorder they should be referred for individualized treatment. In the United States, publicly funded early education intervention programs conduct developmental screening for children three years and younger, the birth-to-three program. When an autism spectrum disorder is recognized these children are legally entitled to therapy. Current approaches, like those that Jeanne Simons pioneered, are incorporated in early intervention programs throughout the United States that recognize the importance of a developmental orientation to treatment.

Current evidence recommends intensive behavioral intervention. Such behavioral programs are being carried out for fifteen hours a week or more on a one-to-one basis for a year or longer using developmental approaches and applied behavioral analysis principles. Such intensive treatment is needed to maximize outcomes. It should begin as early as possible after diagnosis to facilitate the development of communication skills, cognitive functioning, and adaptive behaviors. Applied behavior analysis (ABA) can help children learn new skills through a reward-based motivation system. Many school programs use discrete trial learning (DTT), a structured ABA technique. Discrete trial learning breaks down skills into small, or "discrete," components. These component skills are taught one by one. Parent coaching—teaching parents to use intervention techniques working along with a therapist delivering such behavioral interventions— is important and has been shown to improve outcomes.

Interventions emphasize individualized treatment that focuses on emotional engagement, behavioral supports, and interpersonal approaches that stress intersubjectivity. For example, the Early Start Denver Model (ESDM) is a comprehensive early intervention approach that has been shown effective in controlled clinical trials. ESDM focuses on shared interpersonal engagement in the context of joint attention with positive affect to facilitate an interpersonal sense of "we-ness" and emotional attunement with parent or teacher. This approach seeks to facilitate social communication and language development. ESDM provides a developmentally based curriculum intervention for children with autism twelve to forty-eight months of age (32, 33, 34, 35). The skills to be taught are defined, and teaching procedures are established. ESDM is provided by therapy teams and by parents in group settings or individually, either carried out in the clinic setting or naturalistically integrated into the child's daily home life after school. The ESDM combines a developmentally focused intervention with well-recognized applied behavior analysis procedures.

Paramount to Jeanne Simons' approach is recognition of the perspective of the individual child. At Linwood Jeanne spoke of observing and following each child to learn about him. Current approaches do not necessarily focus sufficiently on taking the time to appreciate the child's preferences to the extent that Jeanne did, for example, in the range of food choices as reinforcers, or in utilizing a child's preferred stereotypy as a reinforcer when selecting reinforcers for behavior. Kanner settled on autistic aloneness and perseverance of sameness as the two core features of autism; *DSM-5* has two parallel diagnostic criteria: persistent deficits in social communication and social interaction, and restrictive patterns of behavior, interests, and activities. In examining a child, I consider both of these sets of criteria, but I think first of Kanner's because they focus on the child's predicament, his sense of social perplexity, and the obsessive desire for sameness and constancy in a confusing world in which he is bombarded by sensory experiences that he must cope with every day.

IN SUMMARY, PSYCHOSOCIAL TREATMENTS are increasingly based on developmental models and behavior analysis. Such treatments are tailored to the needs of individual children. Randomized and large-scale studies are needed to understand and determine the intensity of individualized treatment needed, and to identify the specific symptoms that are responsive to treatment (36). Parental interventions for emotional and behavioral problems are documented to be an essential part of treatment (37).

Studies in targeted subpopulations seek to identify autistic subtypes based on identification of genetic findings or biomarkers with the goal of finding potential new avenues for treatment. Continuing study is needed for medication treatment carried out in the context of defined educational approaches. New approaches are needed for the treatment of co-occurring conditions such as mood disorders. There is no specific drug treatment for autism spectrum disorders. However, adjunctive medication treatment with psychoactive drugs is helpful and has been studied extensively over the years since autism was first described (38, 39, 40). Medication may be needed to address mood disorders and maladaptive behaviors such as aggression, irritability, sleep problems, hyperactivity, inattention, impulsivity, tantrums, and self-injurious behavior. When medications are prescribed they need to be used in conjunction with agreed-upon individualized treatment programs.

Extensive randomized, double-blind placebo-controlled clinical trials, with confirmatory meta-analyses of multiple trials, have identified risperidone and aripiprazole as two drugs with comparable efficacy and safety in pediatric and adolescent patients diagnosed with autism spectrum disorder and co-occurring psychiatric disorders. These two drugs used separately in conjunction with psychosocial treatment are prescribed in the treatment of disruptive behavioral disturbances, including aggression and irritability, hyperactivity/noncompliance, inappropriate speech, and stereotypic behavior (38, 39). The present evidence finds that these drugs are safe, acceptable, and tolerable. Moreover, risperidone has been shown (for example, in a twenty-one-month follow-up continuation following an eight-week placebo-controlled clinical trial) to be safe and efficacious in longer-term treatment of children and adolescents with autism.

When using medications side effects must be closely monitored, because they are commonly observed. For example, increased appetite, weight gain, and enuresis are risks associated with long-term risperidone. These risks must be balanced by longer-term behavioral and social benefits for children.

In addition to advances in diagnosis and classification, better case identification, legal safeguards, genetic studies, and psychosocial and drug treatments, extensive studies in the developmental social and cognitive neurosciences are facilitating early case identification, identifying biomarkers, and mapping brain circuits that may inform future diagnosis and treatments. These neurosciences studies utilize both use rodent animal models and non-human primate models and employ developmental neuroimaging studies in affected children. The Autism Brain Imaging Data Exchange (ABIDE) is a major resource in the study of brain development. These advances are furthered summarized in a seventy-five-year perspective on the growth in knowledge about autism (41).

REFERENCES

1. Bleuler, E. Dementia Praecox or the Group of Schizophrenias. New York: International Universities, 1950 (1911).
2. Kanner, L. Autistic disturbances of affective contact. Acta Paedopsychiatry 1968; 35:100–316. Originally published in The Nervous Child 1943; 2:217–250.
3. American Psychiatric Association. Diagnostic and Statistical Manual of Mental Disorders, 3rd ed. Washington, DC: American Psychiatric Publishing, 1980.
4. American Psychiatric Association. Diagnostic and Statistical Manual of Mental Disorders, 3rd ed. rev. Washington, DC: American Psychiatric Publishing, 1987.

5. American Psychiatric Association. Diagnostic and Statistical Manual of Mental Disorders, 4th ed. Washington, DC: American Psychiatric Publishing, 1994.

6. Asperger, H. "Autistic psychopathy" in childhood. In U. Frith (Ed.), Autism and Asperger Syndrome (pp. 37–92). Cambridge: Cambridge University Press, 1991.

7. Wing, L. Asperger's syndrome: A clinical account. Psychological Medicine 1981; 11:115–129.

8. American Psychiatric Association. Diagnostic and Statistical Manual of Mental Disorders, 5th ed. Arlington, VA: American Psychiatric Publishing, 2013.

9. Moss, J., & Howlin, P. Autism spectrum disorders in genetic syndromes: Implications for diagnosis, intervention and understanding the wider autism spectrum disorder population. Journal of Intellectual Disability Research 2009; 53:852–873.

10. Harris, J. The origin and natural history of autism spectrum disorders. Nature Neuroscience 2016; 26:1390–1391.

11. Frankl, G. Language and affective contact. The Nervous Child 1943; 2:251–262.

12. Baio, J., Wiggins, L., Christensen, D. L., et al. Prevalence of autism spectrum disorder among children aged 8 years—Autism and Developmental Disabilities Monitoring Network, 11 Sites, United States, 2014. Morbidity and Mortality Weekly Report, Surveillance Summaries 2018; 67(6):1–23.

13. Christensen, D. L., Maenner, M. J., Bilder, D., et al. Prevalence and characteristics of autism spectrum disorder among children aged 4 years—Early Autism and Developmental Disabilities Monitoring Network, 7 Sites, United States, 2010, 2012, and 2014. Morbidity and Mortality Weekly Report, Surveillance Summaries 2019; 68(2):1–19.

14. Dunn, D. Public Law 94-142. In F. R. Volkmar (Ed.), Encyclopedia of Autism Spectrum Disorders. New York: Springer, 2013.

15. UN General Assembly. Convention on the Rights of Persons with Disabilities: Resolution adopted by the General Assembly, A/RES/61/106, 24 January 2007. https://www.refworld.org/docid/45f973632.html.

16. Kanner, L. The children haven't read those books: Reflections on differential diagnosis. Acta Paedopsychiatra 1969; 36:2–11.

17. Harris, J. C. The necessity to identify subtypes of autism spectrum disorder. JAMA Psychiatry 2019; 76(11):1116–1117.

18. Weiner, D. J., Wigdor, E. M., Ripke, S., et al. Polygenic transmission disequilibrium confirms that common and rare variation act additively to create risk for autism spectrum disorders. Nature Genetics 2017; 49(7):978–985.

19. Kanner, L. In Defense of Mothers: How to Bring up Children in Spite of the More Zealous Psychologists. Springfield, IL: Charles C. Thomas, 1941.

20. Kanner, L. Infantile autism and the schizophrenias. Behavioral Science 1965; 10:412–420.

21. Fromm-Reichmann, F. Notes on the development of treatment of schizophrenics by psychoanalytic psychotherapy. Psychiatry 1948; 11(3):263–273.

22. Bettelheim, B. The Empty Fortress: Infantile Autism and the Birth of the Self. New York: MacMillan, 1967.

23. Olmsted, D., & Blaxill, M. The Age of Autism: Mercury, Medicine, and a Man-Made Epidemic. New York: St Martin's Press, 2010.

24. Folstein, S., & Rutter, M. Infantile autism: A genetic study of 21 twin pairs. Journal of Child Psychology and Psychiatry 1977; 18:297–321.

25. Huguet, G., Benabou, M., & Bourgeron, T. The genetics of autism spectrum disorders. In P. Sassone-Corsi and Y. Christen (Eds.), A Time for Metabolism and Hormones. New York: Springer, 2016.

26. de la Torre-Ubieta, L., Won, H., Stein, J. L., & Geschwind, D. H. Advancing the understanding of autism disease mechanisms through genetics. Nature Medicine 2016; 22:345–361.

27. Weiner, D. J., Wigdor, E. M., Ripke, S., et al. Polygenic transmission disequilibrium confirms that common and rare variation act additively to create risk for autism spectrum disorders. Nature Genetics 2017; 49(7):978–985.

28. Modabbernia, A., Velthorst, E., & Reichenberg, A. Environmental risk factors for autism: An evidence-based review of systematic reviews and meta-analyses. Molecular Autism 2017; 8(1):13.

29. Lechpammer, M., Wintermark, P., Merry, K. M., et al. Dysregulation of FMRP/mTOR signaling cascade in hypoxic-ischemic injury of premature human brain. Journal of Child Neurology 2016; 31(4):426–432.

30. Simons, J., & Oishi, S. The Hidden Child: The Linwood Method for Reaching the Autistic Child. Baltimore, MD: Woodbine House, 1987.

31. Kanner, L. Childhood Psychosis: Initial Studies and New Insights. New York: John Wiley and Sons, 1973.

32. Rogers, S. J., & Dawson, G. Play and Engagement in Early Autism: The Early Start Denver Model: Vol. 2, The Treatment. New York: Guilford Press, 2009.

33. Dawson, G., Rogers, S., Munson, J., et al. Randomized, controlled trial of an intervention for toddlers with autism: The Early Start Denver Model. Pediatrics 2010; 125:17–23.

34. Rogers, S. J., Dawson, G., & Vismara, L. An Early Start for Your Child with Autism. New York: Guilford Press, 2012.

35. Rogers, S. J., Estes, A., Lord, C., et al. A multisite randomized controlled two-phase trial of the Early Start Denver Model compared to treatment as usual. Journal of the American Academy of Child and Adolescent Psychiatry 2019; 58(9):853–865.

36. Charman, T. Trials and tribulations in early autism intervention research. Journal of the American Academy of Child and Adolescent Psychiatry 2019; 58(9):846–848.

37. Tarver, J., Palmer, M., Webb, S., et al. Child and parent outcomes following parent interventions for child emotional and behavioral problems in autism spectrum disorders: A systematic review and meta-analysis. Autism 2019; 23:1630–1644.

38. Fallah, M. S., Shaikh, M. R., Neupane, B., et al. Atypical antipsychotics for irritability in pediatric autism: A systematic review and network meta-analysis. Journal of Child and Adolescent Psychopharmacology 2019; 29(3):168–180.

39. Aman, M., Rettiganti, M., Nagaraja, H. N., et al. Tolerability, safety, and benefits of risperidone in children and adolescents with autism: 21-month follow-up after 8-week placebo-controlled trial. Journal of Child and Adolescent Psychopharmacology 2015; 25(6):482–493.

40. Maneeton, N., Maneeton, B., Putthisri, S., et al. Aripiprazole in acute treatment of children and adolescents with autism spectrum disorder: A systematic review and meta-analysis. Neuropsychiatric Disease and Treatment 2018; 14:3063–3072.

41. Harris, J. C. Leo Kanner and autism: A 75-year perspective. International Review of Psychiatry 2018, pp. 3–17.

Appendix B
An autism resource guide

When I set out to create a resource guide for parents and caregivers of individuals with autism spectrum disorder (ASD), I did not anticipate that doing so would pose much of a challenge in the age of the internet. What I quickly came to realize, however, was that there is no one site that holds the key to all the financial and educational resources mandated by law and implemented by a large number of agencies across the United States. Neither is there a single source providing comprehensive information about the educational and residential services available to children and teens in every state who cannot be accommodated in public schools.

Thus, what follows is not an exhaustive guide, but it will, I hope, serve as a starting point for the reader seeking ASD resources. It includes the most informative sources I have been able to locate, together with my caveats regarding the limits of the information offered. Federal and state agencies can be contacted through their website or by telephone. The state of Maryland, with which I am most familiar, is my test case to assess the completeness of a site's information.

Publicly funded educational and treatment services for children, teens, and adults with learning disabilities, including ASD, have been mandated throughout the United States since 1975 under PL94-142, revised and renamed in 2004 as the Individuals with Disabilities Education Act (IDEA).

One might logically assume that a list of such services would be available state by state through a central agency, such as the US Department of Health, Education, and Welfare, but **US Facilities and Programs for Children with Severe Mental Illnesses**, the only such compilation I could find that lists all publicly funded services state by state, was published in 1978, with no up-to-date revisions.

Each state's Department of Health provides information about services for children with disabilities, including some listings of preschool and residential educational resources. *Caveat*: Keep in mind that every state uses a different approach to deliver services and may offer differing levels of support. The state's published information may also be incomplete when it comes to specific programs and facilities. In researching the website and subdivisions of the Maryland Department of Health and Mental Welfare, for example, I found that it mentioned only two organizations providing nonpublic services to children and adults with ASD. Calling the state's health department directly may yield better results.

Thirty states have a **specific autism mandate**, which is listed by **the American Speech-Language-Hearing Association (ASHA)** (www.asha .org). These laws and mandates require that every individual receive services in the least restrictive environments, with each state responsible for the delivery of such services.

Medicaid (www.medicaid.gov/medicaid/benefits/autism-services/) specifies the federally mandated autism services that are covered through the Medicaid program.

The National Centers for Disease Control and Prevention (CDC) offers information on some autism treatment modalities, including medication treatment and alternative approaches (www.cdc.gov/ncbddd/au tism/treatment.html).

A number of **private and professional organizations, listed below,** provide information about services for individuals with ASD across the United States.

Easterseals (www.easterseals.com/explore-resources/living-with-autism /state-autism-profiles.html) has the most comprehensive list of agencies that provide services across the fifty states and DC. *Caveat*: The site offers extensive information for each state but few or no specifics about nonpublic treatment centers.

Another Easterseals site (www.easterseals.com/our-programs/autism-services/index.html) outlines the **services** Easterseals itself offers, mainly to young and older adults with autism who are transitioning to more independent living.

Autism Speaks (www.autismspeaks.org) is a national advocacy organization that sponsors research and provides a resource guide for all kinds of services and providers that are "autism friendly," including an **incomplete list of residential programs** across the United States. The organization lists resources by zip code in its guide and has an Autism Response Team (ART). **Autism Speaks** also outlines federal and state disability benefits (www.autismspeaks.org/financial-autism-support), though not state by state. Contact Autism Speaks by email at familyservices@autismspeaks .org and by phone at 888-288-4762.

The **Autism Treatment Network (ATN)** (https://asatn.org/about/loca tions) collaborates with Autism Speaks to provide information about multidisciplinary medical care for children with ASD. It identifies twelve such sites across the United States and Canada.

The **American Academy of Child and Adolescent Psychiatry** (www .aacap.org) has an Autism Spectrum Resource Center. AACAP's information is mainly meant as a resource for physicians and other professionals, but the academy's website lists hospitals and research centers that specialize in the treatment and research of autism.

The **Arc** (www.autismNOW.org) provides a map and directory that lists agencies within each state that can help parents of children with ASD with resources, services, and supplies. *Caveat*: The list does not include a list of local nonpublic schools or residential services for children with autism.

The **Autism Society of America** (www.autism-society.org) provides information about available services across the nation specifically via email through the organization's National Contact Center at info@autism-soci ety.org. The organization staffs a helpline you can call Monday through Friday at 800-328-8476.

The **Autism Society** has **affiliates in every state** that in turn have pull-down menus with information about educational resources and referral services in that state. *Caveat*: I checked out the online information available for Maryland and found that it offered only an incomplete list of nonpublic educational and residential services. If the society is contacted directly with a request for such information, however, it may well be able to provide a more complete listing.

The **American Autism Association** (www.myautism.org) offers mostly information about therapeutic recreational programs and educational resources. Contact the American Autism Association by email at info@my autism.org and by phone at 877-654-4483.

The National Association of Private Special Education Schools (NAPSEC) (www.napsec.org) lists nonpublic schools for children with special educational, developmental, and mental health needs, including children with ASD, in alphabetical order and by state, but its information is incomplete and it does not specify schools that are exclusively geared toward educating students with ASD. For my test case, Maryland, it listed twenty-three schools—a number of which were regional offshoots of the same organization. Of those, only four schools offer services exclusively to children and youth on the autism spectrum, while five included such children among those to whom they cater. Linwood was not on the list.

Recognized Schools for Children with Autism (https://thebestschools.org/features/recognized-schools-for-children-with-autism/) lists thirty-four centers in fifteen states, which means that it leaves out a great number of reputable treatment facilities and schools across the nation.

AngelSense's Autism Schools in USA (www.angelsense.com/blog/autism-schools-in-usa) gets the user to what seems to be by **far the most inclusive list of nonprofit private schools and residential centers for individuals with ASD in the thirty-nine states that appear to have such centers.** *Caveat*: This list, too, is incomplete, listing only four such facilities in Maryland and leaving out Linwood

Every state has a **Parent Training and Information Center (PTI)** (https://www.parentcenterhub.org/find-your-center/) that provides the latest information regarding treatment, education, and research related to ASD.

Under the heading "Autism Spectrum Disorder: Treatment," the **American Speech-Language-Hearing Association (ASHA)** (www.asha.org) offers an exhaustive list of treatment approaches to autism now in use, including applied behavioral analysis (ABA) and the Denver model, used singly or in various combinations. Many of the treatment approaches emphasize parent education (https://www.asha.org/PRPSpecificTopic.aspx?folderid=8589935303&section=Treatment).

Acknowledgments

This book is first and foremost a testament to the indomitable spirit of Jeanne Simons, who dedicated her life to children who, without her, would have ended their lives forgotten in institutions. It is also a testament to friendship. Within the relationship that developed between us, starting with our collaboration on the book *The Hidden Child*, I came to not only admire Jeanne but value her as a friend. And the more I learned about her life the more convinced I became that hers was a story that needed to be told. Had she not come to trust me, she would never have agreed to share it with the world.

At first sight Jeanne was an outgoing, engaging person. In actuality, she was intensely private, and talking about her struggles with her own condition was very difficult for her. But once she had made the decision to do so, she engaged in the project with all of the energy and determination with which she tackled all challenges in her life.

This book would not have seen the light of day without the enthusiastic, active, and patient support of James C. Harris, MD, and his wife, Catherine DeAngelis, MD. The former wrote the very personal foreword and afterword as well as a succinct overview of the history and latest state of knowledge in the field of autism. Catherine, a long-time editor of the *Journal of the American Medical Association*, lent her wisdom to me and her editorial expertise to the manuscript. Together they championed the project and helped it find a publisher. I owe them an immense load of gratitude.

I'm also indebted to Bill Moss, CEO of the Linwood Center until September 2019, who after reading the manuscript recommended it to Dr.

Harris. Bill and his staff have been generous with their time and knowledge, to help me understand what has happened in autism education since I last wrote about it. I think Jeanne would have been proud and pleased with how Linwood has developed under his leadership. With its pioneering past and solid reputation, it will, I hope, survive many more challenges.

I'm grateful to early readers who alerted me to weaknesses in the way the book was originally structured and educated me about modern word usage. I hope I caught all offending anachronisms!

Last but not least, my journey into publishing a book with a university press could not have been made smoother than it was by my editor, Joe Rusko, and his numerous colleagues at Johns Hopkins University Press. A special shout-out to my copy editor, Jackie Wehmueller, whose thoughtful suggestions greatly improved the end product. I emerge unscathed and very grateful that they made it possible for me to deliver on my promise to Jeanne Simons in hopes that her story will inspire and inform a large and diverse readership.

Jeanne Simons, LCSW, ACSW (1910–2005)

Raised and educated in Holland as a certified Montessori teacher, Jeanne Simons worked with unusual children all her life, both in Holland and in the United States. In 1955, she founded the Linwood Children's Center for children with autism in Ellicott City, Maryland. There she pioneered a highly successful treatment approach, described in her book *The Hidden Child: The Linwood Method for Reaching the Autistic Child*, coauthored with Sabine Oishi (1987). Professionals from all over the world came to Linwood to study her methods, and she lectured and consulted in centers in Europe, Japan, and Latin America. It was not until she was middle-aged that she realized she was on the autism spectrum herself.

Sabine Oishi, PhD

Born and raised in Switzerland, Sabine Oishi started out as an elementary school teacher there. After a brief teaching career, she enrolled at the University of Geneva, where she studied child development with the renowned genetic epistemologist Jean Piaget. In the United States she received training in child play therapy and, as part of a doctorate in human development from the University of Maryland, College Park, in family therapy. She worked in both Switzerland and America as a researcher in longitudinal studies about the effects of maternal deprivation and early education (Head Start), respectively, but most of her career was spent as a child, adolescent, and family therapist in community settings. She is the author, with Jeanne Simons, of *The Hidden Child: The Linwood Method for Reaching the Autistic Child* (1987). Sabine may be reached with questions at sabineoishi7@gmail.com.